Env. Pab. Occu. Hlth

D1154873

PATHOLOGICAL EFFECTS OF RADIO WAVES

STUDIES IN SOVIET SCIENCE

PATHOLOGICAL EFFECTS OF RADIO WAVES

M. S. Tolgskaya and Z. V. Gordon
Institute of Labor Hygiene and Occupational Diseases
Academy of Medical Sciences of the USSR
Moscow, USSR

Translated from Russian by
Basil Haigh

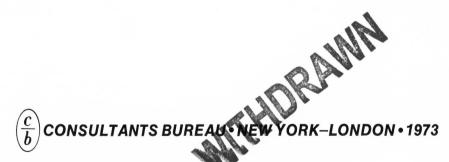

$\frac{c}{b}$ **CONSULTANTS BUREAU • NEW YORK–LONDON • 1973**

AMERICAN MEDICAL ASSOCIATION

LOYOLA UNIVERSITY LIBRARY

Mariya Sergeevna Tolgskaya is head of the Laboratory of Pathomorphology of the Institute of Labor Hygiene and Occupational Diseases of the Academy of Medical Sciences of the USSR. Her main investigations have been devoted to the pathological anatomy of occupational diseases.

Zinaida Vasil'evna Gordon is head of the Laboratory of Radiofrequency Electromagnetic Waves of the Institute of Labor Hygiene and Occupational Diseases of the Academy of Medical Sciences of the USSR. Her main investigations have been devoted to problems of labor hygiene and the biological effects of radiofrequency electromagnetic waves.

(SCI)
QP
341
.T6523
1973

The original Russian text, published for the Academy of Medical Sciences of the USSR by Meditsina Press in Moscow in 1971, has been corrected by the authors for the present edition. This translation is published under an agreement with Mezhdunarodnaya Kniga, the Soviet book export agency.

MORFOFIZIOLOGICHESKIE IZMENENIYA PRI DEISTVII ELEKTROMAGNITNYKH VOLN RADIOCHASTOT

M. S. Tolgskaya and Z. V. Gordon

Морфофизиологические изменения при действии электромагнитных волн радиочастот

Мария Сергеевна Толгская, Зинаида Васильевна Гордон

Library of Congress Catalog Card Number 72-94825
ISBN 0-306-10878-X

©1973 Consultants Bureau, New York
A Division of Plenum Publishing Corporation
227 West 17th Street, New York, N.Y. 10011

United Kingdom edition published by Consultants Bureau, London
A Division of Plenum Publishing Company, Ltd.
Davis House (4th Floor), 8 Scrubs Lane, Harlesden, NW10 6SE, London, England

All rights reserved

No part of this publication may be reproduced in any form without written permission from the publisher

Printed in the United States of America

Envir. Pub. Occu'Hlth.

Contents

AUG 21 1974

SECTION I. Physiological and Morphological
Changes in Animals Exposed to Radio Waves of
High Intensity

SECTION II. Physiological and Morphological Changes in Animals after Prolonged and Repeated Exposures to Low-Intensity Radio Waves of Different Frequencies

Introduction

A large region of the electromagnetic wave spectrum is occupied by electromagnetic waves (or fields) in the radiofrequency band: high frequency (HF), very high frequency (VHF), and super-high frequency or microwave radiation.

The electromagnetic field spreads as electromagnetic waves (radio waves). The wave is formed at a distance greater than its length (λ) from the source, in the wave zone where the electric and magnetic components of the electromagnetic field vary in phase ($E = 377H$) and the emission of energy is measured in terms of the power flux density (PFD) in watts (W/cm^2), milliwatts (mW/cm^2), or microwatts ($\mu W/cm^2$). At a distance less than the wavelength from the source of radiation, i.e., in the zone of induction, the electric and magnetic components (E and H) do not vary in phase, and the emitted energy is evaluated either as the field intensity in volts per meter (V/m) or in amperes per meter (A/m). The energy decreases rapidly with increasing distance from the source (inversely proportional to the square or cube of distance).

Persons working with sources of HF and VHF radiation will evidently be for the most part in the zone of induction, and the intensity of their irradiation may reach thousands of volts and tens of amperes per meter in the HF band (Nikonova, 1963) and hundreds of volts per meter in the VHF bands (Fukalova, 1964, 1968). So far as microwaves are concerned, persons working with microwave generators are as a rule in the wave zone. The intensity of irradiation for them may vary from several microwatts to several milliwatts per square centimeter (Gordon, 1958, 1966). The pres-

1

ence of a wave zone or induction zone under industrial and experimental conditions determines the physical values used to assess
the intensity of irradiation (the power flux density or the field intensity), the instruments used for measuring, and the experimental
technique (irradiation from a distant source, in a cavity resonator,
inductor, capacitor, and so on).

The physical parameters evidently also determine the biological effects of the different frequency bands.

In recent decades various bands of radio waves have been
extensively used in many branches of industry. The microwave
band has been widely applied in the field of radar, radionavigation,
radioastronomy, radiometeorology, radiocommunication, nuclear
physics, and physiotherapy. The short-wave and ultrashort-wave
band are used for physiotherapy, radiocommunication, broadcasting, television, and also for the heat treatment of dielectrics and
for welding plasticized rubber. The long and medium waves are
used for the heat treatment of metals in the vacuum-tube industry
and in mechanical engineering.

In view of the wide use of radio waves in many branches of
industry the study of their biological action on persons working
with sources of radiation requires investigation. A matter of particular importance is the action of radio waves of low intensity,
which are most frequently encountered in industry. Another interesting topic for study is the dynamics of development of pathological changes in the body as the result of prolonged exposure to
low intensities of radiation in the various frequency bands, the
pathogenesis of the lesions, and the mechanism of action of the
radiation. Finally, it is essential to establish maximal allowable
intensities of irradiation for workers exposed to the action of
radiowaves. Earlier investigations have dealt mainly with the study
of high intensities which cause overheating of the body, and it is only
very recently that work has been published which showed that prolonged exposure to low intensities gives rise to certain functional
and morphological changes. Clinical and physiological investigations
have shown that radio waves of low intensity, acting on the human
body, can produce functional changes in the nervous system and,
in particular, in its autonomic division, as well as changes in the
cardiovascular system and neurohumoral disturbances. These
changes have a definite clinical form, and in the overt stages of

the disease it appears as an increasingly severe syndrome of autonomic asthenia, neurocirculatory dystonia, and features of diencephalic insufficiency (Drogichina and Sadchikova, 1968).

Experimental investigations on animals (physiological, biochemical, morphological, etc.) have demonstrated disturbances of activity of the nervous and cardiovascular systems and of metabolism in experimental animals irradiated with radio waves, and the character of the biological effects depends on the intensity and duration of exposure and on the frequency of the waves.

Until now there has been no monograph in either the Soviet or western literature to summarize the morphological and physiological results obtained by experimental studies of the biological effect of radio waves of different intensities.

In this book the authors survey the literature and describe the results of their own morphophysiological investigations, which have extended over many years and have been undertaken with the close collaboration of the Laboratories of Radiofrequency Electromagnetic Waves and of Pathological Anatomy.

The object of these investigations was to discover the general principles governing the development of morphological changes in the organs and tissues of experimental animals exposed to radio waves, to compare them with the functional disturbances, to determine the characteristic features of action of individual wave bands, and to compare the intensity and character of the morphological changes resulting from the action of various frequencies. Besides the study of the biological action of high intensities of radio waves, causing overheating, particular attention has been paid to the action of low intensities of waves in the various frequency bands, not giving rise to a thermal effect, for the reason that the chronic effect of such low intensities is of great importance to persons working under conditions of exposure to radio waves.

The Present State of the Problem

When considering the published material on morphological changes caused by exposure to radio waves it is advisable to examine the available evidence from the standpoint of the general similarities and differences between the biological effects characteristic of the different wave bands. The following two situations

can accordingly be distinguished: the action of high intensities of
irradiation and the action of low intensities, not giving rise to an
integral thermal effect.

Most published work is devoted to the morphological study
of the organs and tissues of animals exposed to the action of short
and, in particular, ultrashort waves (3-300 MHz). The investigators themselves were mainly concerned with discovering whether
such radiation could be used in physiotherapy as a method of deep
heating. This naturally explains the high intensity of the irradiation used in investigations of the biological action of short and
ultrashort waves. In the last decades these frequencies have been
widely used also for radiocommunication, broadcasting, and television purposes, and also in branches of industry using heat treatment of dielectrics, welding of plasticized rubber, and so on. Under
these conditions, despite the high power ratings of the sources of
radiation, the workers using this radiation were exposed to the action as a rule of comparatively low intensities, not sufficient to
raise the body temperature. The short and ultrashort wave bands
are thus interesting as regards the action both of high and, in particular, of low intensities of irradiation.

Microwaves in the 300-300,000 MHz wave band (millimeter,
centimeter, and decimeter waves) have certain special properties
from the physical and health aspects. They differ from radio waves
in the longer part of the spectrum by the limited depth of their
penetration into the body. For example, millimeter waves are absorbed in the surface layer of the skin, centimeter waves at a depth
of 2-4 cm, while decimeter waves penetrate deeper still. From
the health point of view another significant difference is that pos-
sibilities of exposure to microwave irradiation have increased, in
particular with the mass production and exploitation of microwave
generators for use in radar stations, for example. The potential
health hazard of longer radio waves (medium, short, and ultrashort
waves), by contrast with that of microwaves, occurs chiefly in connection with the use of sources of these waves. Microwaves are
important as regards the action of both high and low intensities of
irradiation. Finally, the biological action of the longest radio waves
(long and medium waves of frequencies between 100 kHz and 3 MHz),
despite their extensive use for heat treatment of metals in the vacuum-tube and mechanical engineering industry, has only recently

begun to be investigated. The work of Tolgskaya and Nikonova
(1964) demonstrated for the first time histological changes in the
organs and tissues of irradiated animals exposed to the action of
the electrical and magnetic components of a high-frequency electromagnetic field (medium wavelengths). However, the intensities
of irradiation used experimentally (1800 V/m and 60 A/m) did not
cause an increase in body temperature, and the effect produced was
conventionally regarded as nonthermal.

The morphological picture of changes in the organs and tissues resulting from the action of short and ultrashort waves and
microwaves of high intensity is largely similar in character.

In acute experiments the animals (mice, rats, rabbits) die
quickly with marked evidence of hyperthermia, and in the opinion
of most investigators this is the cause of death, and is indistin-
guishable from the manifestations of ordinary hyperthermia.

Slavskii and Burnaz (1933) and Oettinger (1931), for instance,
observed definite vascular disorders after a single exposure to
short and ultrashort waves: congestion of the brain and internal
organs and multiple petechial hemorrhages in the pleura, pericardium, and meninges. These degenerative changes evidently had no
chance to develop because of the rapid death of the animals and
they were slight in degree. After repeated, brief exposures to
radiation of the same intensity, the vascular disorders and degenerative changes were more severe in character.

Morphological changes accompanying the action of ultrashort
and short waves of high intensities, as Zhukhin (1937), Shibkova
(1937), and others have shown, are characterized not only by hyperemia and hemorrhages in all the viscera and brain, but also by
severe rigor mortis and degenerative changes in the liver cells,
the epithelium of the convoluted renal tubules and the muscle fibers
of the myocardium; degenerative changes also were found in synapses and in nerve cells in various parts of the central nervous system and autonomic ganglia. Acute swelling of the cytoplasm of
nerve cells with vacuolation was particularly marked in the hypothalamic region (Shibkova, 1937; Liebesny, 1936).

Considerable changes are also observed in the gonads,
notably degeneration of the epithelium of the seminiferous tubules
which may progress to their necrosis (Oettinger, 1931; Schliephake,

1932), and degenerative changes in the oöcytes with atrophy of the follicles and cyst formation (Lotis, 1936; Gillerson and Voznaya, 1939).

Morphological investigations of the effects of microwaves until recently consisted principally of studies of the action of centimeter waves, predominantly of high intensity and most frequently emitted continuously. No investigations in the millimeter band could be found in the accessible literature.

Investigations in the 3- to 10-centimeter and decimeter bands (wavelength 21, 40, and 82 cm) undertaken by Milyutina (1938), Seguin and Castelain (1947), Boysen (1953), Pervushin and Triumfov (1957), Dolina (1959), Tolgskaya, Gordon, and Lobanova (1960), Gorodetskaya (1962), Pitenin (1962), and Minecki and Bilski (1961), in which acute experiments were conducted during exposure to high intensities of irradiation, frequently ending in death, revealed marked vascular disorders: congestion, perivascular edema, multiple hemorrhages and numerous infarcts in the lungs, hemorrhages in the spleen, liver, and kidneys. Degenerative changes, just as after irradiation with short and ultrashort waves, evidently had no chance to develop because of the rapid lethal issue.

During chronic exposure, mild congestion of the organs was accompanied by more marked degenerative changes, consisting of swelling of nerve cells in the brain, the appearance of vacuoles in the cytoplasm of individual cells of the hypothalamus, cloudy swelling of the epithelium of the convoluted renal tubules, fatty degeneration of the liver cells, and cloudy swelling and focal homogenization of individual myocardial fibers.

A group of investigations was concerned with the action of high-intensity centimeter waves on the gonads (Imig et al., 1948; Gunn, Gould, Anderson, et al., 1961; Povzhitkov et al., 1961; Bereznitskaya, 1968a,b; Gorodetskaya, 1962, 1963, 1964; Minecki, 1967). With very high intensities of irradiation (250-400 mW/cm^2) third degree burns on the skin of the scrotum and extensive hemorrhages into the testicular tissues were observed. On microscopic examination, coagulative necrosis of the seminiferous tubules was observed. The seminiferous tubules 4 weeks after a single irradiation under these conditions contained no germinative epithelium, and the interstitial tissue contained numerous fibroblasts but few Leydig's cells (Gunn et al., 1961). Irradiation with radio waves can cause irreversible morphological changes in the gonads not only in high intensities, but also in intensities too low to cause body heating. From this point of view the work of Imig et al., who demonstrated morphological changes in the testes which developed at a lower temperature than those caused by convection heating, is of considerable importance.

Other interesting investigations were carried out by Ummersen (1961), who found delay of cell differentiation in the tissues of the developing chick embryo exposed to irradiation of high intensity (400 mW/cm^2).

The results of experimental morphological investigations of the organs and tissues of animals after a single exposure to irradiation by radio waves (short and ultrashort waves, microwaves) of high intensity thus demonstrate the uniform character of the changes observed. These morphological changes are characterized by marked vascular disorders (congestion, perivascular edema, multiple hemorrhages), which are evidently attributable to the thermal effect produced by radio waves of different frequencies. Repeated irradiation leads to more moderate vascular disorders, combined with severe degeneration changes (shrinking and dark staining of the cortical nerve cells, swelling and vacuolation of the cytoplasm of nerve cells, especially in the hypothalamus, cloudy swelling of the epithelium and granular degeneration of the epithelium of the convoluted renal tubules, fatty degeneration of the liver cells, damage to the germinative epithelium, and so on).

Morphological changes produced by the action of low-intensity radio waves have received little attention in the literature.

As has already been stated, Nikonova and Tolgskaya carried out the first investigations into the biological action of medium radio waves at intensities not sufficient to raise the body temperature. Prolonged and repeated (10 months) irradiation of animals (albino rats) in an electric field of intensity 1800 W/m and in a magnetic field of intensity 50 A/m caused moderate histological changes in the animals' organs and tissues. These changes include moderate vascular disorders, changes indicative of irritation of the nervous system in the receptors and synapses, a proliferative reaction of the microglial cells in the brain, and initial degenerative changes in nerve cells of the brain and the viscera.

Investigations into the action of short and ultrashort waves of lower intensities (Slavskii and Burnaz, 1933; Militsina and Voznaya, 1937; Rakhmanov, 1940) demonstrated morphological changes consisting of swelling of the vascular endothelium, especially in the capillaries of the liver, granular degeneration of the epithelium of the renal tubules, irritation phenomena in the spleen (mitoses and the appearance of plasma cells), stimulation of hematopoietic function, and so on. These findings suggest that the reticuloendothelial system participates in the general response of the body to the action of short and ultrashort waves. In response to irradiation with short and ultrashort waves of comparatively low intensities, these workers observed proliferative changes in various organs of the irradiated animals, proliferation of the vascular endothelium, and increase in the number of mitoses and of young cell forms in the bone marrow and spleen, and so on. Vorotilkin (1940) described proliferation of connective-tissue cells and lymphocytes in the liver, myocardium, and lungs of irradiated animals.

There are only isolated reports in the literature of morphological changes caused by microwave irradiation (decimeter, centimeter, and millimeter waves) of low intensity (Gordon, Lobanova, and Tolgskaya, 1955; Pervushin, 1957; Tolgskaya, Gordon, and Lobanova, 1960; Tolgskaya and Gordon, 1960, 1964, 1968). As well as degenerative changes of slight severity, these workers observed a brisk proliferative reaction of the microglia in the brain and reticuloendothelial cells in the viscera. Low intensities of microwave irradiation were found to cause changes in the synapses of the brain and in the receptors of the skin and viscera.

Experimental Material and Method

Since the scope of the investigation covered a wide range of frequencies of radio waves, a number of different sources were used to irradiate the animals.

In the medium wave band animals were irradiated by a generator with frequency 500 kHz to 1.5 MHz, giving an intensity of the electrical component of the field in the capacitor from 0 to 8000 V/m and of the magnetic field in the solenoid from 0 to 160 A/m.

The animals were irradiated with short (14.88 MHz) and ultrashort (69.7, 155, and 191 MHz) waves in cavity resonators

(Figs. 1 and 2). In its construction the cavity resonator consists of a metal box, the size of which is determined by the frequency characteristic of the generator.

In the microwave (decimeter, centimeter, and millimeter waves) band the energy generated was transmitted by horn-type rectangular or conical antennas (Figs. 3 and 4).

Whereas the animals were irradiated with medium, short, and ultrashort waves in closed containers (capacitor, solenoid, cavity resonator), microwave irradiation was given principally from a distance, and the intensity of irradiation was regulated either by changing the distance from the generator or by changing its output power (by means of a power control). In individual cases a contact method was used, so that the microwave energy absorbed in the part of the body irradiated could be estimated.

The animals were mainly irradiated in groups.

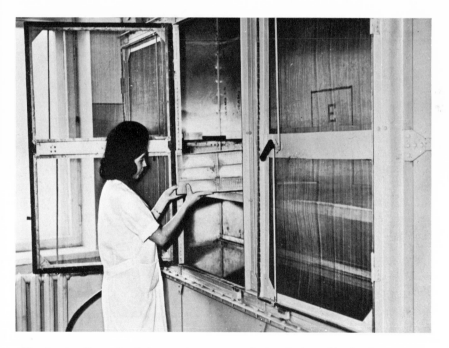

Fig. 1. Loading animals in a cavity resonator for irradiation with ultrashort waves (70 MHz).

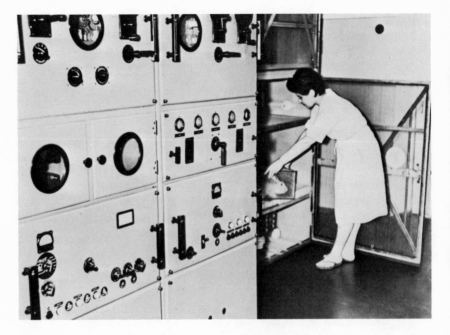

Fig. 2. Preparation of experimental animals for irradiation with short waves (15 MHz).

For irradiation with medium, short, and ultrashort waves the animals were placed in special plastic cages which are virtually transparent to all wave bands and do not cause distortion of the field. For irradiation with microwaves and, in particular, with millimeter waves, the cages were made of polystyrene, with a dielectric constant $\varepsilon = 2.4$-2.9, and with a tangent of the dielectric loss angle of 0.0002-0.0003. By using material of this quality, there was negligible reflection of the waves from the front (irradiated) wall of the cage and losses of energy in the walls were minimal.

The cage with the animals was placed so that the axis of the horn antenna passed through the center of symmetry of the front wall of the cage, which was perpendicular to the axis of the antenna.

The cages for rats contained 6-9 compartments on 2 or 3 levels, while those for mice had 10 compartments on several levels. All cages had ventilating holes in their side walls.

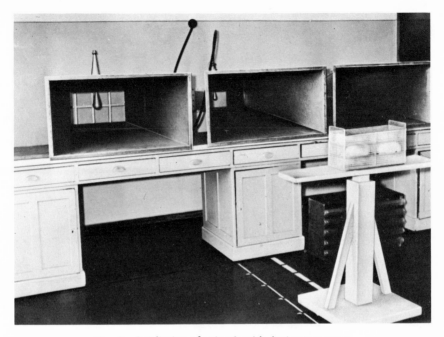

Fig. 3. Irradiation of animals with decimeter waves.

Morphological and physiological investigations were made
on 646 animals (rabbits, rats, mice). Experiments under acute
conditions ranged from a few minutes to 48 h in duration. The experiments with chronic irradiation in low intensities lasted up to
15 months. The animals were killed by decapitation. In the histological investigation, besides ordinary staining methods for the
organs, elective stains were used for the nervous system (central
and peripheral), some histochemical reactions were performed,
and special tests were made of the neurosecretory function of the
hypothalamus and neurohypophysis.

The action of microwaves of the three principal frequency
bands — centimeter, decimeter, and millimeter — was studied sepa-
rately. When a single exposure was used, the microwave intensity
was 40-100 mW/cm^2, and this caused death of the animals. Repeated exposure to high intensities of microwaves also was studied.
The animals were sacrificed 5 months later. With low intensities
of 1-10 mW/cm^2 the duration of irradiation extended up to 10 months.

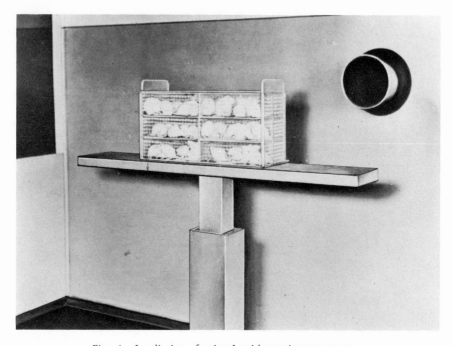

Fig. 4. Irradiation of animals with centimeter waves.

All investigations were carried out in greatest detail using microwave radiation (especially in the 10-cm band). For comparison, and to determine any special characteristics of their action, briefer studies under similar conditions using ultrashort-, short-, and medium-wave radiation are also reported.

Irradiation with ultrashort waves (191, 155, and 69 MHz) was also studied at high (350-5000 V/m) and low (20-150 V/m) intensities; short-wave radiation (14 MHz) was used in high (5000-9000 V/m) and low (2250 V/m) intensities. Irradiation of the experimental animals with medium waves was repeated over a period of 10 months in intensities of 1800 V/m and 50 A/m.

PHYSIOLOGICAL AND MORPHOLOGICAL CHANGES IN ANIMALS EXPOSED TO RADIO WAVES OF HIGH INTENSITY

Introduction

It was decided to describe the material relating to the action of high intensities of radio waves of all frequencies together. The reason for this decision was that the clinical picture of the hyperthermia caused by high-intensity irradiation and the morphological changes are uniform in character.

The clinical picture of hyperthermia in animals irradiated by waves of high intensity is divided into five periods. The first period is that of the usual orienting reaction. In the second and third periods, even if the rat is anesthetized, it awakens. The slight erythema of the paws, tail, and ears in the second period changes into marked hyperemia; the arousal reaction is then followed by depression. In the fourth period the animal is recumbent, clonic convulsions and pareses are occasionally observed, and there is marked hyperemia of the paws, tail, ears, and tip of the nose and edema of the head and genitalia. Finally, in the fifth period the animals lie on their side and there is a copious discharge of blood-stained fluid from the nose and mouth. This period ends with death of the animals followed quickly by rigor mortis.

The duration of each period is determined by the frequency of the waves and the intensity of the irradiation. In the case of short and ultrashort waves and microwaves the first two periods last from 1 to 50 min, the third from 2 to 20 min, and the fourth and fifth from 2 to 30 min.

During irradiation of animals, depending on the intensity of the radiation, changes in rectal temperature may occur in 3 phases (Michaelson et al., 1961a,b; Howland et al., 1961): a slight initial

rise of temperature, followed by a period of equilibrium, and finally a rapid rise of temperature leading to irreversible disturbance
of thermoregulation and death of the animal. However, if the animal is irradiated with microwaves of high intensity ($>100\,\mathrm{mW/cm^2}$
for instance), the maximal rise of temperature occurs sooner and
the animal dies more rapidly. In the investigations described below high intensities of irradiation were used and, as a rule, the
rectal temperature of the animals was found to be increased by
$2-6°C$ (to $42-45°C$). The greatest rise of temperature was observed
in the case of irradiation by 10-cm waves.

Comparison of the level of elevation of the body temperature
during irradiation with waves of equal intensity, for instance with
the shorter microwaves and infrared rays, i.e., in both cases by
radiation which is largely absorbed in the skin, shows that the
microwaves heat the skin more rapidly and to a high temperature,
and death ensues much quicker (Deichman et al., 1959). It thus
appears that the thermal effect is determined not only by the quantity of acting energy, and that even in the case of microwaves of
high intensity, their biological action is not determined entirely by
their thermal effect. This conclusion is very important, becase
later, when the biological action of low intensities of irradiation
(not raising the body temperature) is described, the importance
of low (nonheating) intensities of irradiation in the biological effects
produced by them will also be demonstrated.

Intensities of irradiation giving rise to severe hyperthermia
terminating in death differ for waves of different frequencies.

The way in which the survival period of the animals depends
on the wavelength and intensity of irradiation is shown in Table 1.

Since the intensities of irradiation by waves of different frequencies are expressed in different units, namely, field intensity
or power flux density (volts per meter, milliwatts per square centimeter), the results of the authors' investigations (Gordon and
Lobanova, 1960; Nikonova, 1964; Fukalova, 1964) are given in energy density units (ergs per cubic centimeter). With identical intensities of irradiation by microwaves (100 mW/cm^2 or $33 \cdot 10^{-6}$
erg/cm^3) animals die quickest from the action of 10-cm waves (15
min). With equal intensities of irradiation by ultrashort and short

TABLE 1. Survival of Animals after Irradiation by
Radio Waves of Different Frequencies

Waveband	Intensity of radiation		Time (in min) and percent of animals dying	
	Field intensity and PFD	Energy density in ergs·cm³	50%	100%
Medium (500 kHz)	8 000 V/m	2 830·10⁻⁶	Nil	
Short.	5 000 "	1 100·10⁻⁶	100	
(14,88 MHz)	9 000 "	3 564·10⁻⁶		10
Ultrashort	5 000 "	1 100·10⁻⁵	5	
69.7 MHz.	2 000 "	176·10⁻⁶	100—120	130—200
155 "	700 "	21.5·10⁻⁶	100—120	130—200
191 "	350 "	5.4·10⁻⁶	100—150	160—200
Microwaves				
Decimeter	100 mW/cm²	33·10⁻⁶	60	
Centimeter				
10 cm	100 "	33·10⁻⁶	15	60
3 "	100 "	33·10⁻⁶	110	
Millimeter	100 "	33·10⁻⁶	180	

waves (5000 V/m or 1100·10⁻⁶ erg/cm³) animals exposed to ultrashort waves die within 5 min and those exposed to short waves after 100 min. In the medium-wave bands irradiation at 8000 V/m
did not cause death of the animals for many hours, whereas irradiation in the short-wave band at 9000 V/m caused rapid death (10 min)
of all the animals (100%).

Hence, with a decrease in wavelength the energy density (ED)
causing death of the animals decreases down to the microwave range
and then rises slightly. Whereas medium waves with ED = 2830·
10⁻⁶ do not cause death of animals over a period of many hours,
short and ultrashort waves with much lower ED values (176·10⁻⁶
to 5.4·10⁻⁶ erg/cm³) lead to death of 50% of the irradiated animals
at about the same times (after 100-120 min).

In the case of microwaves with equal ED, 50% of the animals
die after times varying from 15 to 180 min. The 10-cm waves have
a particularly rapid action and the clinical picture of the hyperthermia is very severe.

Let us consider the morphological changes in the organs of
four groups of animals exposed to irradiation by waves of different
frequencies (microwaves, ultrashort, short, and medium waves).

Morphological and Physiological Changes Following Exposure to High-Intensity Microwaves (Centimeter, Millimeter, and Decimeter Bands)

Morphological Changes Following Exposure to High-Intensity Centimeter Waves

Morphological changes were investigated after a single exposure to 3-cm and 10-cm waves of high and medium intensities, causing phenomena of hyperthermia in animals.

The results showed that exposure to 3- and 10-cm waves is accompanied by functional and morphological changes.

The material can be divided into groups depending on the intensity of irradiation and the period of exposure. Since the morphological changes in the animals within each group were identical, the results will be described for groups as a whole.

G r o u p 1. After a single (25-40 min) exposure of animals to 3-cm and 10-cm waves of high intensity (40-100 mW/cm^2), severe clinical manifestations of hyperthermia terminating in death were observed.

Autopsy revealed severe vascular disorders, in the form of hyperemia and multiple hemorrhages in the brain and meninges, the peritoneum, the pleura, and the pericardium. Rigor mortis was severe. Microscopic examination revealed vascular disorders

in the nervous system and viscera, in the form of hyperemia, perivascular edema, and multiple small hemorrhages in the brain,
myocardium (Fig. 5b,c), pleura, epicardium, and intestinal mucosa.

The vascular disorders were accompanied in the brain by
edema of the oligodendroglia, with the appearance of drainage forms
(Fig. 6b,c), acute swelling of nerve cells in different parts of the
brain with solitary vacuoles in the cytoplasm of individual neurons
(Fig. 7b), by homogenization and sometimes by fatty degeneration
of single fibers of the myocardium (Fig. 8b,c), and by changes in
the testicles, in which albuminous masses were deposited in the
lumen of individual tubules and, in some cases, necrosis of single
seminiferous tubules was observed (Fig. 9b). In every case the
content of ribonucleoproteins was reduced in the epidermis and in
its derivatives in the upper layers of the skin. Cloudy swelling
was observed in the epithelium of the convoluted renal tubules and
there was fatty degeneration of the liver cells. There was a total
absence of proliferative response of the microglia in the brain and
of the reticuloendothelial elements in the liver. This protective,
adaptive response is suppressed by irradiation with high-intensity
radio waves of various frequencies.

Group 2. The animals were irradiated once (for 30 min)
with pulsed 10-cm waves with an intensity of 20 mW/cm^2. There
were no deaths among the animals, which were sacrificed immediately after the end of irradiation showing slight signs of hyperthermia. Autopsy showed that the vascular disorders were not
as severe as in the preceding group. Well-marked rigor mortis
was found.

Histological examination showed acute swelling of nerve cells
in various parts of the brain, with solitary vacuoles in the cytoplasm,
swelling and homogenization of the muscle fibers of the myocardium, and initial degenerative changes in the form of cloudy swelling of individual hepatocytes and epithelial cells of the convoluted
renal tubules, against the background of vascular disorders. There
was no proliferative reaction of the microglia in the brain and no
proliferation of reticuloendothelial elements in the liver.

After a single exposure of the animals to pulsed 3-cm waves
for 30 min at an intensity of 20 mW/cm^2, as a rule no evidence of
hyperthermia was observed. None of the animals died. All were
sacrificed immediately after the end of irradiation.

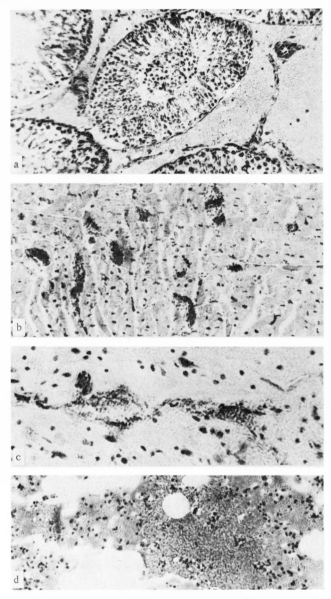

Fig. 5. Comparative characteristics of vascular disorders after single exposure to high-intensity irradiation with waves of different frequencies. Hematoxylin-eosin: a) multiple hemorrhages in stroma of testis following exposure to millimeter waves, 400 ×; b) multiple hemorrhages in myocardium after exposure to centimeter waves, 200 ×; c) multiple hemorrhages in brain after exposure to decimeter waves, 200 ×; d) multiple hemorrhages in lumen of alveoli following irradiation by short waves, 160 ×.

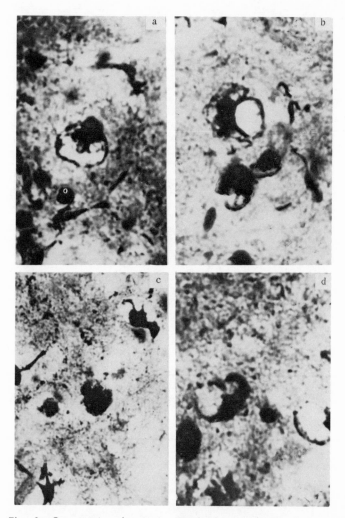

Fig. 6. Comparative changes in oligodendroglia after irradiation
by high-intensity waves of different frequencies. Stained by Miyagawa–Aleksandrovskaya method, 600×: b and c) edema of individual oligodendrogliocytes with formation of "drainage cells."
Irradiation by centimeter waves: a and d) edema of individual
oligodendrogliocytes with the formation of "drainage cells" (a, irradiation by millimeter waves; d, irradiation by decimeter waves).

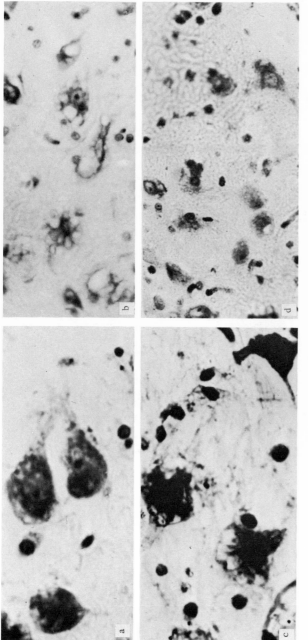

Fig. 7. Comparative effects on nerve cells of the hypothalamic region of irradiation by high-intensity waves of different frequencies. Stained by Nissl's method: a) vacuolation of hypothalamic nerve cells after irradiation with millimeter waves, 630 ×; b) vacuolation of hypothalamic nerve cells after irradiation with centimeter waves, 570 ×; c) vacuolation of hypothalamic nerve cells after irradiation with decimeter waves, 630 ×; d) vacuolation of nerve cells and swelling of their cytoplasm after irradiation with short waves, 320 ×.

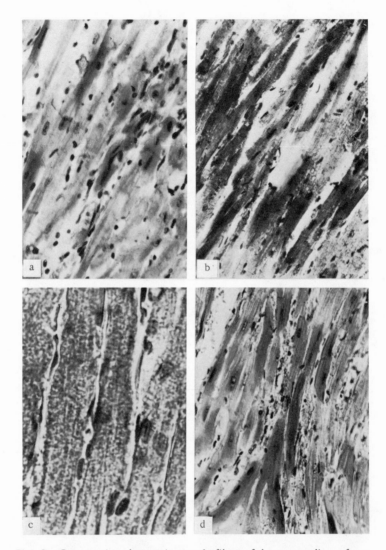

Fig. 8. Comparative changes in muscle fibers of the myocardium after
irradiation by high-intensity radio waves of different frequencies: a) unevenness of staining of muscle fibers after irradiation with millimeter
waves. Hematoxylin-eosin, 330×; b) well marked unevenness of staining and homogenization of myocardial muscle fibers after irradiation with
centimeter waves. Hematoxylin-eosin, 330×; c) fatty degeneration of
myocardial muscle fibers after irradiation with centimeter waves. Sudan
III, 660×; d) homogenization and unevenness of swelling of myocardial muscle
fibers after irradiation with decimeter waves. Hematoxylin-eosin, 330 ×.

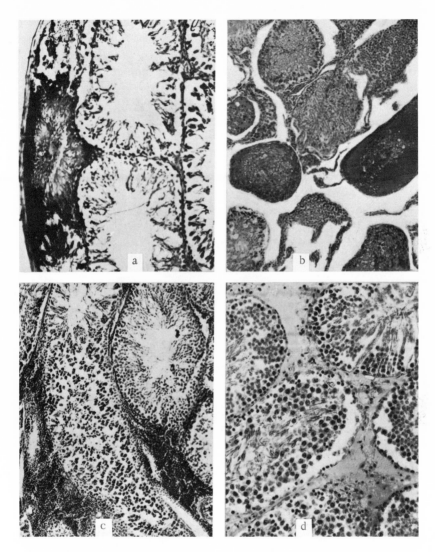

Fig. 9. Comparison of changes in testes after irradiation of high-intensity radio waves of different frequencies. Hematoxylin-eosin: a) necrosis of a tubule beneath the capsule, 330×; b) deposition of albuminous masses in lumen of individual seminiferous tubules and necrosis of tubules in the testis after irradiation with centimeter waves, 280×; c) multiple hemorrhages in testis after exposure to decimeter waves, 330×; d) edema of testicular stroma of animal irradiated with ultrashort waves, 450×.

Histological examination revealed slight hyperemia, perivascular edema in the brain, and swelling of the cytoplasm of the nerve cells with single tiny vacuoles, congestion and swelling of individual muscle fibers of the myocardium, with unevenness of their staining, and also congestion and slight cloudy swelling of the cytoplasm of the hepatocytes and epithelial cells of the convoluted renal tubules. Hyperemia and edema were present in the intestine, spleen, lungs, and testes. Comparison of the effects of pulsed 3-cm and 10-cm waves demonstrates that the 10-cm waves produce the more marked changes.

Group 3. Morphological changes in the viscera and nervous system were studied in 75 albino rats exposed repeatedly (75 sessions) to pulsed and continuous irradiation with 10-cm waves and pulsed 3-cm waves of high intensity (40 mW/cm^2) but with a very short duration of irradiation (5-10 min).

Severe clinical manifestations of hyperthermia were observed in the animals only in the first sessions of irradiation. Later they tolerated the irradiation satisfactorily, their body temperature returned to normal, and the gain in weight of the young experimental animals was the same as in the controls. The animals were decapitated after 75 sessions of irradiation. At autopsy a varied degree of hyperemia was found. Rigor mortis was not so evident as in the preceding groups. The liver was flabby and yellow in color. The kidney tissue was dull, with a slightly swollen cortical layer.

Histological examination of the organs and tissues of the animals sacrificed immediately after repeated irradiation revealed moderate vascular disorders in the brain and viscera. Degenerative changes, in the form of shrinking and dark staining of individual cortical neurons and swelling of the cytoplasm with lysis of the tigroid substance and the appearance of small vacuoles in individual cells of the hypothalamus, were observed in the brain cells. Swelling, unevenness of staining, and homogenization were found in individual groups of myocardial fibers, occasionally they showed fatty degeneration, and there was slight fatty degeneration also of individual hepatocytes. A brisk proliferative response of the microglia was present in the brain (Fig. 14a) and proliferation of the reticuloendothelial elements in the liver (Fig. 14b), i.e., a brisk proliferative reaction of the reticuloendothelial elements participating in both local and general protective and adaptive reactions of the body. In all irradiated animals the degenerative changes in the nervous system and viscera described above were focal in character and cells of normal configuration could always be seen side by side with pathologically changed cells.

Although the irradiated animals had slight degenerative changes in the viscera and nervous system, together with ill-defined vascular disorders, they remained apparently healthy during their period of survival, reflecting the well-developed compensatory powers of the body as a whole.

The next step was to investigate morphological changes in particularly sensitive structures of the nervous system. For this purpose, changes were studied in the receptors of the skin and interoceptors in various receptive fields of the viscera in 25 animals (rabbits and rats) after irradiation with 10-cm waves of high intensity.

Changes in the skin receptors were particularly interesting because during exposure of the living body to radio waves the skin is the first barrier which they meet. Because of its rich supply of afferent nerve endings the skin is a powderful receptive field, whose response to the action of radio waves largely determines the response of the body as a whole. It was no less interesting to determine changes in the interoceptors of the viscera for, according to published observations, the interoceptors of the viscera are very sensitive to various harmful agents, even of minimal character.

In recent years Lavrent'ev's school has amassed an extensive material on the morphology and pathology of the sensory innervation of the viscera. They have shown that sensory fibers participating in the innervation of the viscera arise from neurons of the spinal and, sometimes, of the cranial ganglia.

Interoceptors of the viscera help to maintain the relative constancy of the internal medium which is a condition of the normal existence of the organism. If, however, stimulation is excessive, pathological changes may arise. Chernigovskii states that resonance arising in the nervous system due to stimulation of receptive fields embraces very many physiological processes. In other words, stimulation arising from interoceptive fields disturbs the activity of the somatic muscles, the smooth muscles, the res-

piratory, circulatory, and hematopoietic systems, and the work of
the kidneys and adrenals, and it upsets metabolism.

According to Chernigovskii, this wide irradiation is a characteristic feature of stimulation from interoceptors in general,
and from vascular interoceptors in particular.

Many different workers have studied changes in the interoceptor system of the viscera in diseases and during exposure to harmful factors. They have studied changes in the interoceptor system
of several reflexogenic zones: 1) the gastrointestinal tract, 2) the
periendomyocardium, 3) the arch of the aorta, carotid sinus, and
walls of large blood vessels. Investigations have been made in
patients with cancer, peptic ulcer, intestinal obstruction, hypertension, diphtheria, tuberculosis, and uremia, and subjects exposed
to ultrahigh-frequency and x-ray irradiation and to experimental
anoxia (Dolgo-Saburov; Kupriyanov; Lavrent'ev; Plechkova). Morphological changes thus revealed in receptors of the various receptive fields were basically similar and consisted essentially of
irritation phenomena and degenerative changes expressed to different degrees.

Changes in the interoceptors resulting from exposure to
superhigh-frequency radiation were studied by Pervushin (1957),
who showed that reversible and irreversible changes take place
in the interoceptors of the heart under these conditions.

According to Pervushin, superhigh-frequency irradiation
acts primarily on afferent fibers of the spinal ganglia, and changes
in the peripheral components of the autonomic nervous system are
slight in degree.

In the present investigation no encapsulated or free nerve
endings were found. Mainly thin afferent (sensory) nerve fibrils
of the skin and viscera were studied. The fact that these fibrils
belonged to sensory (afferent) fibers in every case was proved by
their origin from myelinated nerve trunks (traced by the study of
serial sections). The object of the investigation was to show changes
in afferent nerve fibrils of the skin and viscera during irradiation,
and whether these were "boutons terminaux," preterminals, or
larger sensory nerve fibrils was of no fundamental importance.

To begin with the receptor system of the viscera and skin
was studied in 10 healthy control animals from which pieces of the

receptive (reflexogenic) zones were taken: from the skin of the
ear and thigh, the urinary bladder, esophagus, stomach, intestine,
atrium, and arch of the aorta.

Examination of all the material showed, more so in some
cases than in others, thin, delicate myelinated nerve fibers enter-
ing the smooth muscles or connective tissue of an internal organ
or the epithelium of the skin, dividing into small twigs branching
in different directions and having the appearance of delicate, thin
fibrils. Sensory nerve fibrils were then investigated in the various
receptive fields of the viscera and skin of animals irradiated with
centimeter waves of different intensities.

At the same time, nerve cells of the spinal sensory ganglia
(cervical, thoracic, lumbar, and sacral), the autonomic ganglia
(solar plexus, ganglia of the vagus nerve), and of the hypothalamic
region were investigated in the same animals.

Considerable changes were found in the sensory nerve fibers
in the receptive fields of animals sacrificed immediately after a
single exposure to irradiation with pulsed 10-cm waves of high
intensity, ranging from 40 to 100 mW/cm^2, for 15 min. Since the
changes in the nerve fibers of the different receptive fields were
more or less identical as a manifestation of the nonspecific response of the body, and the only differences were in the degree of
their intensity, they will be described collectively. First, in all
the viscera and skin investigated, nerve fibrils were more numerous than in the control animals, a result which can evidently be
explained by the increased argyrophilia of the nerve fibrils of these
receptive fields and their better impregnation with silver. Increased argyrophilia of the afferent nerve fibrils is evidence of
their irritation. Frequently strongly argyrophilic, black, swollen
fibrils with irregular swellings, pools of axoplasm, and even fragmentation were seen (Figs. 10c and 11a). The thin sensory nerve
fibrils were on the whole affected to an equal extent in all the receptive fields investigated, but comparison of the changes in the
sensory nerve fibrils of the viscera and skin revealed that those
in the skin were most severely affected, the lesion involving a
larger number of nerve fibrils and the changes being more severe
in character, sometimes involving fragmentation of the fibrils.

Swelling of the cytoplasm and lysis of the tigroid substance
in the center of the cell, with ectopia of the nucleus, were found

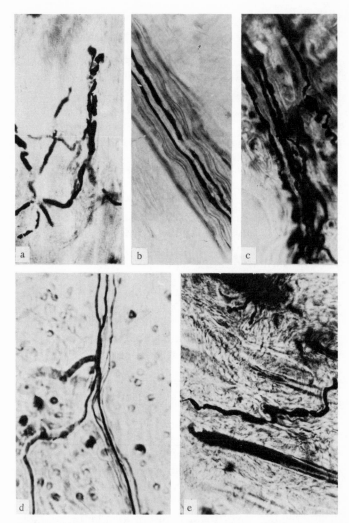

Fig. 10. Comparison of changes in sensory nerve fibers of receptive fields of the skin
after irradiation by high-intensity waves of different frequencies. Bielschowsky—Gros.
a) Thickened myelinated cutaneous nerve fibers, with increased argyrophilia, breaking
up into fragments after irradiation with millimeter waves, 400 ×; b) axons of myelinated cutaneous nerve fibers (large myelinated trunks) are strongly argyrophilic and have
irregular swellings, with fragmentation in some places, after irradiation with millimeter
waves, 350 ×; c) very marked argyrophilia, irregular swellings, tortuosity of cutaneous
nerve fibers after irradiation with centimeter waves, 400 ×; d) delicate network of thin,
unchanged cutaneous fibers after irradiation with decimeter waves, 400 ×; e) increased
argyrophilia and irregular swellings of cutaneous nerve fibers after irradiation by short
waves, 400 ×.

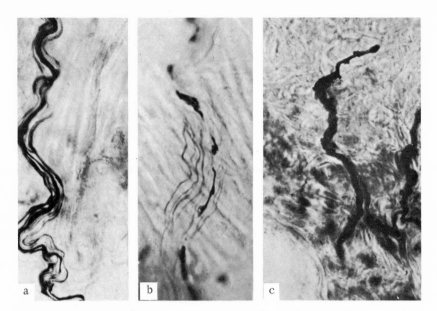

Fig. 11. Comparison of changes in sensory nerve fibers of viscera after irradiation by high-intensity waves of different frequencies. Bielschowsky–Gros. a) Very marked argyrophilia with irregular swellings of a myelinated nerve fiber of the atrial myocardium after irradiation with centimeter waves, 440×; b) side by side with thin, delicate fibers, a strongly argyrophilic fiber, breaking up in some places into fragments, is seen in the urinary bladder after irradiation by decimeter waves, 600×; c) very marked argyrophilia, irregular thickening of sensory nerve fibers in the myocardium after irradiation by ultrashort waves, 440×

in the nerve cells of the spinal sensory ganglia. Some cells were seen with swollen cytoplasm containing tiny vacuoles. Signs of karyocytolysis and death of individual neurons were observed. The nerve cells of the autonomic ganglia were only slightly altered.

With all intensities of irradiation the worst affected structures were the small sensory fibrils, i.e., the preterminal portions of the receptor system, and the larger afferent fibrils, in agreement with the findings of Dolgo-Saburov, Kupriyanov, and Pervushin, who regard the preterminal portions of the afferent fibers as the most vulnerable.

The changes discovered in the sensory nerve fibers of the receptive fields of the viscera and skin following exposure to centimeter waves are not specific. Similar changes have been found

by other workers (Lavrent'ev, Plechkova, Falin, Vyropaev, Guseinov, Rakhmatullin, Alekseev, etc.) in various diseases and after
exposure to various harmful agents.

As was mentioned above, after irradiation with centimeter
waves of high intensity the damage of the sensory fibrils of the
skin was particularly severe and the degenerative changes in those
fibrils progressed as far as fragmentation of individual fibrils.
The reason for this may be that the skin is the first barrier in the
path of the radio waves, and part of the energy which falls on it is
absorbed by it.

Parallel with the changes in the sensory nerve fibers of the
skin, after irradiation with centimeter waves histochemical changes
were studied in the skin itself. The content of ribonucleoprotein
(RNP) in the skin of the irradiated animals was determined by
Brachet's reaction. The results showed a decrease in the RNP
content in the epidermis and its derivatives and, in particular, in
the surface layers of the skin (Fig. 13b).

When the morphological changes observed in animals exposed
to pulsed and continuous 10-cm waves were compared, they were
found to be more severe after exposure to the pulsed waves.

Comparison of the morphological changes observed after
exposure to 10-cm and 3-cm waves of high intensity showed that
they were more severe after exposure to the 10-cm waves.

Morphological Changes Following Exposure to High-Intensity Millimeter Waves

Half of the animals receiving a single exposure to millimeter
waves with an intensity of 100 mW/cm^2 for 180 min died 3 h after
the end of irradiation with evidence of marked hyperthermia. The
other half of the animals were sacrificed with a similar clinical
picture. At autopsy severe congestion and small hemorrhages
were found in the brain and viscera. Rigor mortis was very pro-
nounced.

On histological investigation of the organs of these animals,
marked vascular disturbances were present, evidently associated
with the hyperthermia. They consisted of severe hyperemia of
the viscera and brain, perivascular edema, and multiple small
hemorrhages in the brain, myocardium, liver, kidneys, mucous

membrane and submucosa of the intestine and pancreas, beneath
the capsule and the stroma of the testes (Fig. 5a), and in the lumen
of the alveoli. Acute swelling and a few vacuoles also were found
in the hypothalamic nerve cells (Figs. 7a), together with edema
of the oligodendroglia with the formation of "drainage" cells (Fig.
6a), irregular staining and homogenization of myocardial muscle
fibers (Figs. 8a), edema of the testicular stroma, necrosis and
homogenization of solitary seminiferous tubules, particularly those
located beneath the capsule (Fig. 9a), swelling of the epidermis
of the skin, and edema and hyperemia of the dermis.

Histochemical investigation showed a decrease in the RNP
content in the cells of many visceral organs and of the nervous system.
However, these changes were most conspicuous in those organs
which normally have a high RNP content in the cytoplasm of their
cells. These include: nerve cells, the glandular epithelium of the
gastrointestinal tract and pancreas, the epithelium of the bronchi
and trachea, cells of the secondary follicles of the spleen, the
endothelium of the capillaries, the ependyma of the ventricles of
the brain, and the epidermis of the skin and its derivatives. The
changes in RNP content varied from slight pallor of the cytoplasm
to its complete transparency. Cells of the epidermis of the skin
and its derivatives were particularly severely affected (Fig. 13a).

The content of deoxyribonucleoproteins (DNP) in the viscera
was more stable. Only very slight changes were found in the DNP
content in the cell nuclei of tissues affected by cloudy swelling
(hepatocytes, epithelium of the convoluted renal tubules, spermatogenic epithelium of the testes) and in the hypothalamic nerve
cells with signs of karyocytolysis.

A special feature of the changes in RNP content in the cells
of the epidermis and its derivatives in the skin should be emphasized. The changes in the derivatives of the epidermis diminished in intensity toward the deep layers of the skin.

Changes in the sensory nerve fibers of the receptive fields
of the skin were very severe. They took the form of argyrophilia
and the appearance of beads and pools of axoplasm, or in some
cases, fragmentation of the cutaneous nerve fibrils (Fig. 10a). Increased argyrophilia and irregular swellings were found even in
fibers of the large myelinated trunks in the dermis (Fig. 10b).
Nerve fibrils of the receptive fields of the viscera (myocardium,

aorta, esophagus, intestine, stomach) were much less severe and
signs of irritation were found. If the animals survived for a long
period after irradiation, cloudy swelling was observed in the epithelium of some convoluted renal tubules and hepatocytes, and in
a few cases there was fatty degeneration of the hepatocytes and the
epithelium of a few convoluted renal tubules.

Animals exposed to a single irradiation with millimeter
waves in an intensity of 140 mW/cm^2 for 15 min did not die. Signs
of hyperthermia were observed, but they were less marked than
in the preceding group. In all the viscera, the skin, and the nervous system, histological examination revealed vascular disorders
less severe than in the preceding group, but still of considerable
intensity. Acute swelling of the nerve cells was found in the
brain, especially in the hypothalamus, with the appearance of solitary vacuoles in their cytoplasm and occasionally with signs of
karyocytolysis. Unevenness of staining and homogenization of the
myocardial muscle fibers, edema of the stroma and homogenization of individual seminiferous tubules (necrobiosis), subcapsular
hemorrhages in these organs, cloudy swelling in the epithelium
of the convoluted renal tubules and, to a lesser degree, in the
hepatocytes, and slight thickening of the alveolar septa through
hyperemia and edema were found. After irradiation in an intensity of 40 mW/cm^2, changes also were found in the sensory nerve
fibers of the cutaneous receptive fields. The fibers were strongly
argyrophilic and had irregular swellings and pools of axoplasm
on them. The sensory fibrils of the viscera were relatively unchanged. Nerve cells of the spinal sensory ganglia, just as after
irradiation with 10-cm waves in an intensity of 100 mW/cm^2,
showed swelling of the cytoplasm in individual cases, with lysis of the
tigroid substance in the center of the cell and ectopia of the nucleus.
Phenomena of karyocytolysis with death of individual neurons (Fig.
12) were evident. Since millimeter waves are absorbed by the skin,
the changes in the nerve cells of the spinal ganglia can be attributed only to reflex mechanisms.

Histochemical tests showed a decrease in the RNP content,
especially in the cells of the epidermis and its derivatives in the
skin. The decrease in RNP content in the viscera was much less
marked.

The DNP content in the cell nuclei of the viscera was unchanged, but in the nuclei of the epidermis it was considerably

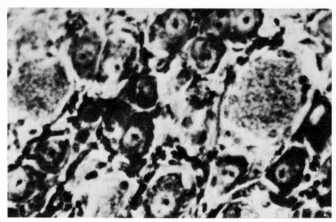

Fig. 12. Swelling of cytoplasm with tigrolysis and ectopia of the nucleus in some cells, and with evidence of karyocytolysis and death of the neurons in other cells in a spinal ganglion after irradiation with millimeter waves in high intensity. Nissl's stain, 450×.

reduced. A decrease in the DNP content was also observed in foci of cloudy swelling in the hepatocytes and epithelium of the convoluted renal tubules and also in the nerve cells of the hypothalamic region showing signs of karyocytolysis.

Morphological Changes Following Exposure to High-Intensity Decimeter Waves

The animals were irradiated with decimeter waves in an intensity of 100 mW/cm^2 for 60 min; 50% of the animals died with manifestations of hyperthermia.

Macroscopic examination revealed clearly defined features of hyperthermia in all the animals, in the form of vascular disorders (very marked congestion of the viscera and brain) and rigor mortis. Microscopically, evidence of perivascular edema and multiple small hemorrhages were found in the brain (Fig. 5c) and also in the liver, lungs, myocardium, and stroma of the testes (Fig. 9c).

Against the background of the vascular disorders, acute swelling of the brain neurons was observed, together with the appearance of solitary large vacuoles in the hypothalamic nerve cells (Fig. 7c), edema of the oligodendroglia (Fig. 6d), and swelling and

homogenization and unevenness of staining, and sometimes fatty
degeneration of the myocardial muscle fibers (Fig. 8d). Slight
cloudy swelling was seen in the hepatocytes and the epithelium of
the convoluted renal tubules.

Changes in the sensory nerve fibers in various receptive
fields of the viscera (myocardium, aorta, esophagus, intestine,
stomach, urinary bladder, etc.) were very marked. The changes
consisted of argyrophilia of the nerve fibrils, tortuosity, the appearance of beads and pools of axoplasm, and sometimes fragmentation of individual nerve fibers. However, no damage was found
to the sensory nerve fibers of the skin. They were thin and delicate,
and they had no swellings or pools of axoplasm (Fig. 10d).

Histochemical tests showed a decrease in the RNP content
in the cytoplasm of cells of the viscera and nervous system, more
conspicuous in organs normally rich in RNP (nerve cells, glandular
epithelium of the gastrointestinal tract and pancreas, bronchial
epithelium). The RNP content in the skin was not reduced (Fig.
13c).

Considerable vascular disorders were found in the testes, in
the form of edema of the stroma and small hemorrhages beneath
the capsule and in the stroma of the organ.

*   *   *

Comparison of the morphological changes found in the animals after exposure to microwaves of all frequencies in high intensity shows that these changes were uniform in character, i.e.,
they were due mainly to the thermal action of the radiation.

High intensities of irradiation with microwaves of different
frequencies caused death of the animals with clinical features of
severe hyperthermia. The morphological changes in the tissues
and organs of the irradiated animals consisted of severe vascular
disorders, acute swelling and vacuolation of the cytoplasm of the
nerve cells in various parts of the brain, and unevenness of staining, homogenization, and fatty degeneration of the myocardial fibers.
However, despite the fact that the thermal effect masked all the
finer changes, this does not mean that all the changes can be
ascribed to the thermal effects alone. Exposure to microwaves gives
rise to some phenomena of a special kind. For example, despite
the high intensity of irradiation with decimeter waves, the sensory

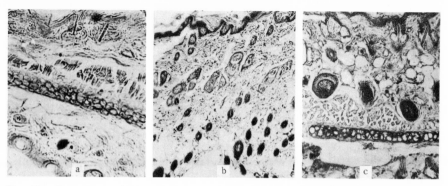

Fig. 13. Comparison of histochemical changes in the skin (RNP content) after irradiation by waves of different frequencies in high intensity. Brachet's reaction: a) sharp decrease in RNP content in epidermis and its derivatives in top layers of skin with integrity of RNP in epidermal derivatives in deeper layers of the skin after irradiation with millimeter waves. 120×; b) decrease in RNP content in epidermis and its derivatives in upper layers of skin with integrity of RNP in epidermal derivatives in deeper layers of the skin after irradiation with centimeter waves. 200×; c) normal content of RNP in epidermis of skin and its derivatives after irradiation with decimeter waves. 160×.

nerve fibrils of the skin were unchanged. Yet, at the same time, they were severely affected by exposure to centimeter and, in particular, to millimeter waves. This difference can be explained by the fact that millimeter waves are absorbed by the skin, and most of their effects are observed on the skin and its sensory nerve fibers (the other changes in the viscera are evidently reflex in character). This was also confirmed by the clearly defined changes in the nerve cells of the spinal sensory ganglia, which showed evidence of irritation (swelling, central tigrolysis of the cytoplasm, and ectopia of the nuclei). Although after exposure to microwaves of various frequencies and of high intensity the differences between the morphological pictures were thus apparently masked, it must be noted that the 10-cm waves gave rise to the severest effects, for death took place earlier, the picture of hyperthermia was more marked, and the vascular disorders were more extensive. Second place in order of severity of effects was occupied by the decimeter waves, and third place by millimeter waves.

The intensity of the biological action of microwaves is determined by the intensity and frequency of the waves and the duration of exposure to them.

Without dwelling in detail on the biological effects of high-intensity irradiation (measured in hundreds of milliwatts per square centimeter), it will merely be noted that such intensities lead to severe hyperthermia and, if the exposure is long enough, to death. The morphological changes in the tissues and organs of the animals consisted of severe vascular disturbances, accompanied by less marked degenerative changes in the nervous system and viscera, presumably on account of the earlier death of the animals. No proliferative reaction of the microglia was observed in the brain or of the reticuloendothelial elements in the viscera. This protective and adaptive reaction was evidently inhibited by the effects of the high-intensity microwaves. This pattern is characteristic of the whole band of microwaves and is due to their considerable heating effect.

Millimeter waves, which are absorbed completely in the skin and act on its sensory nerve fibers, irritating them and sending an intensive flow of impulses along the afferent fibers to the spinal ganglia and on into the brain, have a lower thermal threshold. However, if the irradiation is of high intensity (40 mW/cm^2) the dynamics of the temperature response is such that the integral heating effect is more marked in the case of centimeter waves. These waves, which are absorbed only partially in the skin and which penetrate deeper, evoke a well-defined temperature response to irradiation of high intensity evidently as a result of their direct action on the tissues and on the thermoregulatory centers.

So far as decimeter waves are concerned, they are virtually unabsorbed in the skin and penetrate deeper into the body, where they evoke a thermal effect if the PFD levels are high.

Morphological Changes in Animals Following Exposure to Ultrashort Waves (69.7, 155, and 191 MHz) of High Intensity

After a single exposure to ultrashort waves (69.7 MHz, intensities 5000 and 2000 V/m) the animals died with well marked features of hyperthermia. At autopsy severe hyperemia and small hemorrhages were found in the brain and viscera, with well-developed rigor mortis. Microscopic investigations shown marked vascular disturbances in the brain and viscera, with hyperemia and perivascular edema in the lungs, brain, and liver, edema of the myocardial and testicular stroma, and multiple perivascular hemorrhages in the brain, lungs, liver, kidneys, myocardium, and testes. Because death occurred quickly (5 min after irradiation in an intensity of 5000 V/m), degenerative changes had not had time to develop in the viscera and they were slight in degree. Acute swelling of the cytoplasm was observed in the nerve cells in various parts of the brain. After irradiation with ultrashort waves in an intensity of 2000 V/m the animals survived rather longer (up to 3 h), and the picture of vascular disturbances as described above was accompanied by degenerative changes in the nerve cells of the brain and viscera which were rather more clearly defined, and consisted of swelling and vacuolation of the cytoplasm of nerve cells in the thalamus and hypothalamus. Marked argyrophilia and irregular swellings and pools of axoplasm were found in the sensory nerve fibers of the skin and sensory fibrils of the myocardium, intestine, urinary bladder, esophagus, and elsewhere (Fig. 11c).

Homogenization and unevenness of staining of the myocardial muscle fibers, swelling of these fibers (with edema of the stroma), and cloudy swelling with, occasionally, fatty degeneration of the hepatocytes and epithelium of the convoluted tubules were found.

Animals irradiated with ultrashort waves with a frequency of 155 MHz and intensity of 1000 V/m and with a frequency of 191 MHz and intensities of 700 and 350 V/m died 17-200 min later (depending on the intensity of the irradiation) with marked features of hyperthermia. Changes similar to those described above, but more severe, were found.

Hence, after exposure to high intensities of ultrashort waves (5000, 2000, and 1000 V/m) with frequencies of 69.7, 155, and 191 MHz, death quickly ensued; the animals showed marked evidence of hyperthermia and severe vascular disorders (hyperemia, perivascular edema, and multiple hemorrhages). The vascular disorders provided a background for ill-defined degenerative changes in the nerve cells of the brain, the muscle fibers of the myocardium, and other parenchymatous organs.

If the animals survived longer (up to 3 h), vascular disturbances in the nervous system and internal organs were similar to those described above, and they were accompanied by more definite degenerative changes in the nerve cells, and marked signs of degeneration of sensory nerve endings in the skin and viscera. Degenerative changes were found in the muscle fibers of the myocardium, the spermatogenic epithelium of the testes, the hepatocytes, and the epithelium of the convoluted renal tubules.

Morphological Changes in Animals Exposed to Short and Medium Radio Waves of High Intensity

G r o u p 1. After a single exposure to irradiation with high-intensity (9000 and 5000 V/m) short waves the animals died with signs of marked hyperthermia in 10-1000 min. At autopsy congestion of the brain and meninges and focal hemorrhages in the brain and meninges and in the serous membranes were found. Rigor mortis was severe.

Microscopic investigation revealed considerable vascular disturbances in the brain and all the viscera: congestion, stasis, perivascular edema, and multiple small or larger perivascular hemorrhages in the brain, kidneys, liver, and lungs. Hemorrhages into the lumen of the alveoli also were present in the lungs (Fig. 5d).

If death took place early, the degenerative changes in the nerve cells and viscera were slight in degree. If the animals survived longer, the vascular disturbances were marked and were accompanied by acute swelling of nerve cells in various parts of the brain, with vacuolation of the cytoplasm in the hypothalamic neurons (Fig. 7d).

The sensory nerve fibrils of the viscera and skin showed marked argyrophilia and irregular swelling in different receptive fields (Fig. 10e). Homogenization and unevenness of staining were found in the muscle fibers of the myocardium. Cloudy swelling and, sometimes, fatty degeneration affected individual groups of hepatocytes and epithelial cells of the convoluted renal tubules.

Consequently, after irradiation with short waves of high intensity (9000 and 5000 V/m), leading to death in 10 to 100 min with well-marked evidence of hyperthermia, acute and severe vascular disturbances can be detected morphologically in the nervous system and viscera and are accompanied by ill-defined degenerative changes in the nerve cells, the muscle fibers of the myocardium, and other internal organs. Evidence of irritation of cutaneous sensory nerves and of sensory fibrils of the viscera is clearly visible.

After irradiation with high intensities of short and ultrashort waves the differences between the morphological picture associated with the action of each particular frequency disappear. Everywhere vascular disturbances are predominant, with ill-defined degenerative changes and irritation of sensory nerve fibers of the various receptive fields of the skin and viscera.

However, the impression is obtained that the changes are more severe and developed earlier in the case of irradiation with ultrashort waves. This correlates with the clinical evidence of earlier death after irradiation with ultrashort waves.

Group 2. Irradiation with medium waves with an intensity of 8000 V/m. With waves of this length it was impossible to obtain intensities sufficiently high (even in the case of long or repeated exposures) to cause fatal hyperthermia, because the field voltages of up to 8000 V/m which were used were only on the threshold for producing a thermal effect. The effects of waves of these frequencies will accordingly be discussed in the section on the chronic action of low intensities not inducing a thermal effect.

Comparison of Morphological Changes Following Exposure to Radio Waves of High Intensity and of Different Frequencies

Morphological changes associated with exposure to micro-waves and ultrashort, short, and medium radio waves can be use-fully compared.

In the first series a morphological study was made of the organs and tissues of animals (305) irradiated with radio waves of high intensity and of various frequencies: a) microwaves with intensities of between 40 and 100 mW/cm^2, b) ultrashort waves with intensities of 5000 and 2000 V/m; c) short waves with intensities of 9000 and 5000 V/m. The animals of all groups died with marked signs of hyperthermia. At autopsy, rigor mortis was severe. The rectal temperature of the cadaver as a rule was very high, some-times reaching 40-44°C. The nasal mucosa were cyanosed, and the skin of the paws, ears, and tail strongly hyperemic. Marked con-gestion of the brain and meninges and petechial hemorrhages be-neath the serous membrane of the intestine, the pleura, and the peri-cardium, and in the gastric mucosa and the meninges and brain tis-sues were found. The brain tissue was congested and edematous. The liver was severely hyperemic, and sometimes had an icteric tinge. The spleen was severely congested, and dark liquid blood exuded from its cut surface. The kidneys were congested and flab-by and the capsule stripped easily.

Microscopic investigation showed considerable vascular changes in the nervous system and viscera: severe hyperemia, marked perivascular edema, and multiple small hemorrhages in the stroma of the testes, brain, myocardium, lungs, liver, kidney, and intestinal wall (Fig. 5a,b,c,d). Severe hyperemia and edema in the brain affected both the brain tissue and the meninges; stasis and perivascular and pericellular edema were evident. Changes in the oligodendroglia consisted of edema and the formation of drainage cells (as described by P. E. Snesarev), which are associated with the presence of acute vascular disturbances accompanied by cerebral edema and disturbances of water and mineral metabolism (Fig. 6a,b,c,d).

Damage to the central nervous system was the most conspicuous feature. In sections stained by Nissl's method and by the histochemical reaction for ribonucleoproteins, changes were found in nerve cells in various parts of the brain, more especially in the hypothalamus. Acute swelling of the cytoplasm of the neurons was accompanied by tigrolysis and by a sharp decrease in the ribonucleoprotein content. In animals which survived longer, tiny vacuoles appeared in the cytoplasm of the swollen nerve cells, and their contest gave a negative reaction for lipids (Fig. 7a,b,c,d).

Similar changes (vascular disorders and degenerative changes in nerve cells) took place in the spinal cord and spinal sensory ganglia, and were much less marked in the autonomic ganglia.

After the central nervous system, the myocardium was next most severely affected. Microscopic examination of the heart muscle showed unevenness of staining of the myocardial muscle fibers: some fibers stained very intensely, homogeneously, and had lost their cross-striation, while others, on the other hand, were pale with a distinct cross-striation. Sometimes fatty degeneration of individual muscle fibrils was observed (Fig. 8a,b,c,d). Next in order of severity of damage were the testes. Congestion and edema of the interstitial tissue were clearly defined. Degeneration of the spermatogenic epithelium and, sometimes, necrosis of the tubules or the liberation of albuminous masses into the lumen were observed in individual seminiferous tubules, most frequently those situated beneath the capsule (Fig. 9a,b,c,d).

Congestion and perivascular edema were very evident in the lung tissue, and here and there small perivascular hemorrhages

and hemorrhages into the lumen of the alveoli could be seen (Fig. 5d).
Sometimes there was focal edema of the alveoli, associated with focal
emphysema. The liver tissue was severely hyperemic and sometimes
edematous; the structure of the hepatic columns was disturbed, and
Desse's spaces were widened. The hepatocytes were swollen, with
palely stained nuclei and granular cytoplasm. Side by side with
these cells, others with darkly stained cytoplasm could be seen.
In the kidneys severe hyperemia and perivascular edema were accompanied by tiny perivascular hemorrhages and well-marked evidence of cloudy swelling in the epithelium of the convoluted tubules.
Hyperemia in the spleen was severe, with obliteration of the pattern of the follicles.

It must be emphasized that after a single exposure to radio
waves of high intensity no proliferative response of the microglia
in the brain or of the reticuloendothelial elements in the liver was
observed. This protective and adaptive response was evidently
inhibited by the action of the high-intensity radio waves.

The differences between the morphological picture associated
with the action of radio waves of different frequencies tended to be
obliterated in the case of high-intensity irradiation. Vascular disturbances in the nervous system and viscera dominated the pathological picture.

Compared with the vascular disturbances, the degenerative
changes in the nervous system and viscera were not so clearly
defined. This was probably because they had not had time to develop because of the early death of the animals, and the usual morphological methods were unable to reveal them clearly. However,
some morphological differences between the effects of individual
frequencies of radio waves could be identified. For example, after exposure to millimeter and centimeter waves necrosis of individual seminiferous tubules located beneath the capsule was most
frequently observed (Fig. 9a,b), while after exposure to decimeter
and ultrashort waves the testicular damage was more uniformly
distributed and vascular disturbances in the tissues of the testes
were predominant (Fig. 9c,d).

More precise histological methods (elective staining of nerve
tissue and investigation of receptors) and histochemical methods
revealed more distinct changes in the nervous system and viscera.
Sensory nerve fibers of various receptive fields (skin of the ear

and thigh, the myocardium, aorta, esophagus, intestine, stomach, and urinary bladder) showed definite signs of irritation as reflected by marked argyrophilia, irregular swellings and pools of axoplasm, or even fragmentation of the fibrils (Fig. 10a,b,c,d,e).

Characteristic differences between the effects of different wave bands were also clearly revealed by a study of the lesions of the sensory nerve fibers in the different receptive fields. After exposure to centimeter and, in particular, to millimeter waves the severest changes took place in the cutaneous sensory nerve fibers (Fig. 10a,b,c), whereas after exposure to decimeter waves the cutaneous sensory nerve fibers were unchanged (Fig. 10d), but by contrast the sensory nerve fibrils of the viscera were most severely damaged by the action of decimeter waves (Fig. 11b).

Simultaneously with the sensory nerve fibers in the various receptive fields of the skin and internal organs, changes were studied in the spinal sensory ganglia, where the nerve cells showed central tigrolysis of the cytoplasm and ectopia of the nuclei. Sometimes signs of karyocytolysis were present, with death of individual neurons (irradiation with centimeter, decimeter, and ultrashort waves). Changes were found in the neurons of the spinal sensory ganglia after irradiation with millimeter waves (Fig. 12). Since millimeter waves are absorbed in the skin, changes in the neurons of the spinal ganglia are evidently reflex in origin.

Histochemical investigations revealed a decrease in the content of ribonucleoproteins in the cytoplasm of the cells of many internal organs and of the nervous system. The content of deoxyribonucleoproteins was more stable.

Histochemical changes were more severe in the skin (decrease in the ribonucleoprotein content in the epidermis and its derivatives), especially after exposure to millimeter and centimeter waves, but not after exposure to decimeter waves (Fig. 13a, b,c).

Comparison of the morphological changes found in animals exposed to radio waves of all these frequencies and of high intensity confirms, and this must be stressed repeatedly, that when high intensities of irradiation are given the morphological changes are virtually uniform in character and are associated primarily with the thermal effect.

However, some characteristic differences can be found as a result of exposure to the different wavelengths, and these can be attributed to the characteristic action of the waves rather than to hyperthermia. For example, after exposure to millimeter waves the sensory nerve fibers of the skin are particularly severely affected, and they exhibit well-defined histochemical changes, whereas after exposure to decimeter waves the skin is almost unaffected. The skin is also damaged by the action of ultrashort and short waves.

Exposure to decimeter waves leads to the severest changes in the sensory nerve fibers of the viscera.

A group of animals was also exposed for a short time (5 min) to irradiation by high-intensity (40 mW/cm^2) radio waves in the 10-cm band, which was repeated altogether 75 times.

The animals tolerated the first exposures to irradiation badly. Their body temperature rose sharply, they developed erythema of the limbs and ears, and they lay on their sides. All these phenomena disappeared after 2-3 h. After the subsequent exposures the animals showed less marked effects. In animals sacrificed after 75 exposures (immediately after the last irradiation) vascular disturbances were found but they were only slight by comparison with those in the groups of animals receiving lethal irradiation. The rigor mortis also was not so severe. However, microscopic investigation showed hyperemia and edema of the brain, the lungs, the interstitial tissue of the myocardium, the kidneys, and liver. The vascular disturbances were accompanied by degenerative changes which were most marked in the nervous system, myocardium, and testes. Shrinking of the cortical nerve cells was accompanied by acute swelling of the cytoplasm of nerve cells in the thalamus and hypothalamus, with tigrolysis and vacuolation. Sensory nerve fibers in the skin and viscera showed considerable changes consisting of marked argyrophilia, and irregular beading of the individual fibrils or their complete fragmentation. In this group of animals, by contrast with the group exposed to acute lethal irradiation, a proliferative response of the microglia in the brain and of the reticuloendothelial elements of the viscera was observed (Fig. 14a,b). This is evidence of a protective and adaptive response.

Accompanying the vascular disturbances, there were changes in the muscle fibers of the myocardium, the staining of which was

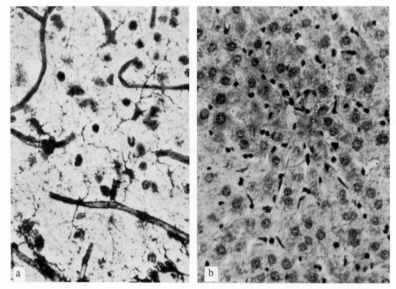

Fig. 14. Proliferative changes in the microglia of the brain and reticuloendothelial elements of the liver after irradiation by high-intensity waves: a) proliferation of microglia around the cerebral vessels after repeated irradiation with
centimeter waves. Miyagawa—Aleksandrovskaya's stain, 325×; b) proliferation
of reticuloendothelial elements of the liver after repeated irradiation with centimeter waves of high intensity. Hematoxylin—eosin, 325×.

visibly uneven. Some fibers were dark, homogeneous, swollen,
and without their cross-striation while others were pale and thin.
Cloudy swelling and fatty degeneration of individual fibers were
present.

Considerable changes were found in the testes. Individual
tubules showed degenerative changes of the spermatogenic epithelium with desquamation of the epithelium into the lumen, and
occasionally with necrosis of individual tubules. However, side
by side with these changes in individual tubules, in most tubules
of the testes evidence of spermatogenesis was clearly visible.
These observations regarding testicular damage following repeated
irradiation by radio waves do not agree fully with those described
by other workers (Imig, Gunn, et al.), who report inhibition of
spermatogenesis in irradiated animals.

Conclusion

Comparison of the morphological changes arising after exposure not only to microwaves of various frequencies, but also to longer radio waves (ultrashort, short, and medium), shows that in the case of the acute action of high intensities of radio waves of whatever length, because of the early death of the animals and the sharp predominance of vascular disturbances, differences between the morphological changes in the organs and tissues of the irradiated animals are to a large extent obliterated. Nevertheless, it is possible to distinguish, when comparing the effects of high-intensity radio waves of different frequencies, that centimeter waves give rise to the most marked effects: the hypothermic manifestations are particularly severe and death takes place sooner. Second place is occupied by decimeter waves, and third place by the shortest bands of ultrashort and short waves. Next follows the band of millimeter waves. The last place is occupied by medium waves, which, even in comparatively high intensities, do not cause hyperthermia or death of the animals. The changes discovered in the animals are principally attributable to hyperthermia. However, although the thermal effect masks the finer changes, not all the changes discovered after exposure to high intensities of radio waves can be attributed entirely to the thermal effect.

Individual changes (changes in the sensory nerve fibers of the skin and viscera, histochemical changes in the skin) indicate that radio waves of different frequencies, but of high intensity, differ in their effects. For example, after exposure to decimeter waves the sensory nerve fibers of the skin are unchanged, and sensory nerve fibers of the viscera are more severely damaged, whereas after exposure to millimeter waves the sensory nerve fibers of the skin suffer particular damage and the sensory nerve fibers of the viscera are only slightly affected. Sensory nerve fibers of the skin and viscera are about equally affected by irradiation with ultrashort, short, and centimeter waves.

PHYSIOLOGICAL AND MORPHOLOGICAL CHANGES IN ANIMALS AFTER PROLONGED AND REPEATED EXPOSURES TO LOW-INTENSITY RADIO WAVES OF DIFFERENT FREQUENCIES

AMERICAN MEDICAL ASSOCIATION

Introduction

In the preceding section it was shown that the effects of radio waves are predominantly thermal and that there are certain characteristic differences between the effects of irradiation by high-intensity radio waves of different frequencies.

However, both in industry, during high-frequency heat treatment of metals and dielectrics, and also in radio communication (broadcasting and television), radar, etc., despite the high output ratings of the transmitters used, persons working with them as a rule run the risk of exposure to irradiation at intensities too low to produce a thermal effect.

To avoid differences of interpretation, the term "thermal effect" will be taken to imply the presence of an integral thermal effect, defined as the temperature response of a human or animal subject.

As the authors showed in 1957 for centimeter waves, and later for other bands, intensities of irradiation not sufficient to induce a thermal effect are by no means inactive on the living organism.

Chronic exposure to low intensities often gives rise to functional changes which may vary in their severity. This conclusion has been reached after many years of experimental study of integral parameters such as the ability of animals to tolerate irradiation, changes in the body weight, the temperature response, and so on, and reactions of systems which are sensitive to the energy of radio waves. These functional changes may affect the nervous and cardiovascular system and metabolism, and they may be accompanied by morphological changes.

The biological action of radio waves of different frequencies is on the whole consistent in direction.

The functions investigated and the character of the changes observed during long-term experiments on animals by Bereznitskaya, Gordon, Zepina, Kitsovskaya, Lobanova, Nikogosyan, Tolgskaya, and Fukalova are given in Table 2.

However, there are certain specific differences between the biological effects of different wave bands. These differences are due to differences in the severity, the time of appearance, and the character of the course of the animal's response to the various frequencies of waves. In the first place certain integral indices characterizing the response of the organism as a whole to radio waves of nonthermogenic intensities and of different frequencies will be described.

Investigations (Gordon, Lobanova, Nikonova, Fukalova) have shown that radio waves of different frequencies have different thresholds of their thermal effect. The highest intensities of irradiation not giving rise to a thermal effect are given in Table 3. Since the units of measurement of intensity of irradiation differ for waves of different lengths, the results are also given in the table as common units of energy density (ergs/cm^3).

It will be clear from Table 3 that as the wavelength shortens, the energy density values for which there is no increase in body temperature fall steadily, except in the ultrashort wave band. No explanation for this phenomenon can yet be given. It can only be assumed that the special behavior of the ultrashort wave band is due to a resonance effect in heterogeneous structures and macromolecules (Bach et al., 1961; Cook, 1952; Moskalenko, 1960; Franke, 1960).

Allowing for these maximal values associated with absence of an integral thermal effect, an experimental study was made of the chronic action of radio waves of different frequencies on animals. The dynamics of body weight was used as the integral index of biological action of the radio waves.

TABLE 2. Functions Investigated and Character of
Changes Observed

Function investigated	Character of changes
Integral indices	
Tolerance	Lowered
Weight	Lowered
Central nervous system	
Conditioned-reflex activity	Weakening of excitation and increase in limiting inhibition in the CNS
Strong acoustic stimulation of rats particularly sensitive to ringing of a bell	Lowering of excitability and weakening of fundamental nervous processes
Electroencephalography	Lowering of bioelectrical activity, and, in some cases, appearance of epileptoid responsiveness to sensory provocation
Cholinergic processes	
Cholinesterase	Lowering of activity of CNS
Acetylcholine	Increased content in CNS
Nicotine-like cholinergic receptors	Lowering of excitability
SH-groups	Reduced content in brain stem
Biochemical changes	
Proteins and protein fractions	Decrease in content of globulin fractions in blood serum
Nonprotein nitrogen	Reduced content in blood
Amino acids	Reduced content in urine
RNA	Reduced content in spleen, liver, and brain
Ascorbic acid	Reduced content in brain stem and increase in adrenals and spleen
Histamine	Increased content in blood, fluctuating changes
Vascular tone	Hypotensive effect
Circulating blood	Tendency toward leukopenia, changes in myeloid series (decrease in number of polymorphs)

TABLE 2 (Continued)

Function investigated	Character of changes
Sexual function	
Ovarian function	Disturbance of estrous cycle
Fertility	Reduced in irradiated females, tendency toward postmaturity, stillbirth
Progeny	Retardation in development, high postnatal mortality
Eyes	Retinal angiopathy, cataract

TABLE 3. Intensity of Irradiation Not Raising Body Temperature

Wave band	Threshold of non-thermal effect	Energy density, in ergs/cm^3
Medium (500 kHz)	Below 8 000 V/m	2 830·10^{-6}
Short (14.7 MHz)	2 250 "	224·10^{-6}
Ultrashort.		
69.7 MHz.	150 "	0.995·10^{-6}
155 "	50 "	0.11 ·10^{-6}
191 "	20 "	0.018·10^{-6}
Microwaves:		
decimeter.	Above 40 mW/cm^2	13.2 ·10^{-6}
centimeter (3 and 10 cm). . . .	10 "	3.3 ·10^{-6}
millimeter	7 "	2.31·10^{-6}

There is reason to suppose that the deviation in weight of the
irradiated animals (mice) is largely determined by the intensity of
irradiation and, to some extent, also by the frequency of the waves.
Low intensities of irradiation in the ultrashort wave band, according
to some investigators, stimulate the animals' gain in weight, but
the majority consider that the gain in weight is retarded (Golysheva
and Andriyasheva, 1937; Skipin and Baranov, 1934; Glezer, 1937;
Voznaya and Zherdin, 1937; Derevyagin, 1939; Tikhonova, 1948).
As regards the superhigh-frequency band, only a few isolated papers
have been published (Denier, 1933; Kutting, 1955; Gordon, Lobanova,
and Tolgskaya, 1955; Lobanova, 1960). They indicate that prolonged
exposure to an SHF field stimulates gain in weight. Finally, radia-

tion in the medium wave band, according to Nikonova, causes no changes in the pattern of gain in weight by irradiated animals.

Changes in weight of animals exposed to radiation in different wave bands (from data obtained by Gordon, Lobanova, Nikonova, and Fukalova) are shown in Table 4. In every case intensities of irradiation not giving rise to an integral thermal effect (not causing an increase in the rectal temperature) were used.

The results given in this table show conclusively that any decrease in the amount of weight gained by the experimental animals compared with controls and the degree of that difference are definitely connected with wavelength.

Centimeter waves have the strongest action in depressing development of the animals (the increase in weight and the time when the increase begins to diminish compared with the control). With an increase in wavelength (decimeter, ultrashort, short waves) this inhibitory effect weakens. It is low at the extreme limits of the radio wave spectrum (millimeter and medium waves), but in the millimeter band the difference arises much later than in other bands (starting with the third month of irradiation) and the greatest decrease is observed after 6 months (when the weight is 45 g less than in the control series).

TABLE 4. Changes in Weight of Animals Exposed
to Radio Waves of Different Lengths

Wave band	Intensity of irradiation	Beginning of change (mos. irradiation)	Gain in weight of animals, in g (mean value)	
			irradi-ated	control
Millimeter	10 mW/cm^2	3	65	75
Centimeter				
3 cm	10 "	1	42	70
10 "	10 "	1.5	25	70
Decimeter	10 "	2	95	120
Ultrashort				
191 MHz	20 V/m	2.5	125	145
155 "	50 "	3.5	110	128
69.7 "	150 "	4	182	210
Short	2 250 "	4	180	210
Medium	1 800 "	10	No change	
	50 A/m	10	"	"

In the medium wave band the difference between the gain in weight of the irradiated and control animals was not statistically significant.

Consequently, the dynamics of the body weight, as an index of development of the animals, is to some extent dependent on the wave band of the radiation.

The effect of radio waves on vascular tone in man and experimental animals has frequently been demonstrated.

Without discussing in detail the responses arising in man to radio waves of different frequencies, it will suffice to mention that in the high-, ultrahigh-, and superhigh-frequency bands a hypotensive effect has been described in workers with radio frequency generators by investigators who have observed mainly vagotonic responses, with a tendency toward hypotension (Parin and Davydov, 1940, 1959; Osipov, 1953; Abrikosov, 1958; Sadchikova and Orlova, 1958; Orlova, 1960; Obrosov and Yasnogordoskii, 1961; Smurova, 1962).

Experimental investigations on animals, undertaken at the Institute of Work Hygiene and Occupational Diseases, Academy of Medical Sciences of the USSR, to study the action of radio waves of different frequencies (Gordon, 1960, 1964; Nikonova, 1964; Fukalova, 1968) have shown that chronic exposure to radio waves of nonthermogenic intensity causes a persistently low blood pressure. This is often preceded by a phase of raised pressure (Table 5).

Although a persistent decrease in blood pressure is a common feature after exposure to radio waves of all frequencies, each individual wave band is associated with its own characteristic changes:

1. Absence of the first phase — elevation of the pressure — in animals irradiated with medium, 3-cm, and millimeter waves;
2. The rapid appearance of the first phase (first week of irradiation) in the case of irradiation with decimeter and 10-cm waves;
3. Early appearance of the second phase of lowering of pressure after irradiation in the ultrashort (69.7 MHz) and short wave bands in the 6th week of irradiation;

TABLE 5. Changes in Blood Pressure After Irradiation with Radio Waves

Wave band	Intensity of irradiation	First phase - elevation of pressure (weeks)	Second phase - pressure reduction (weeks)	% pressure decrease
Medium (500 kHz)	1 800 V/m	Not significant		
	5 A/m	—	30	11.7
Short (14.8 MHz)	2 250 V/m	2	6	12
Ultrashort				
69 7 MHz	150 "	2	6	17
155 "	50 "	2	12	33
191 "	20 "	4	12	29
Microwaves:				
decimeter	10 mW/cm²	1	10	17
centimeter				
10 cm	10 "	1–6	22	11
3 "		—	6	25
millimeter	10 "	—	4	20

4. A considerable (20–33%) decrease in the blood pressure level, especially after irradiation by waves in the millimeter, 3-cm, and ultrashort (155 and 191 MHz) wave bands.

Great importance is attached to the hypothalamus in the mechanism of autonomic vascular disturbances.

Results obtained in the writers' laboratory indicate that the diencephalon is concerned in the response of the body to irradiation with radio waves. Zenina investigated brain potentials and showed that the effects of cardiazol, which evokes paroxysmal responses of diencephalic origin, are inhibited or totally suppressed by microwave irradiation. In this case it can be assumed that the action of the microwaves was to block particular areas of the diencephalon.

Disturbance of hypothalamic activity after exposure to radio waves has also been observed when the effects of microwaves on specialized forms of appetite and electrolyte metabolism were studied in irradiated rats. Hypothalamic nuclei form the higher center for the control of water and mineral metabolism. Kulakova (1968) found no correlation between the intensity of certain types of salt appetite and the electrolyte composition in the body. This could possibly have been due to a disturbance of the mechanism controlling the distribution of salts and water between the cell and the internal medium.

Evidence of the important role of the hypothalamus is given by the clinical picture of the severe forms of disturbances arising after chronic exposure to radio waves, characterized by the diencephalic syndrome (Drogichina and Sadchikova, 1964). This syndrome is manifested as paroxysmal states resulting from neurocirculatory disorders. Distinct disturbances of cortical electrical activity are present.

As a vital part of the brain the hypothalamus plays an important role in the integration of nervous and humoral processes. The hypothalamus can regulate, in particular, the activity of the cardiovascular system, the content of mediators such as acetylcholine, cholinesterase, and histamine, and so on.

Recent investigations undertaken at the Institute of Work Hygiene and Occupational Diseases have shown that radio waves, especially microwaves, can affect certain cholinergic processes. Clinical observations show that chronic exposure to microwaves leads to functional disturbances of the nervous system. The most characteristic disturbance affecting the autonomic nervous system is a tendency for parasympathetic control over the cardiovascular system to predominate. An investigation of neurohumoral regulation (Nikogosyan) revealed an increase in the acetylcholine content in the CNS and a decrease in cholinesterase activity and in the content of SH-groups in the brain stem (Kitsovskaya).

Kitsovskaya (1968) showed that exposure to microwaves lowers the excitability of nicotine-like cholinergic receptors, while the state of the muscarine-like cholinergic receptors remains unchanged. Changes in the state of the former may be to some extent responsible for the disturbance of transmission of excitation in the CNS. The absence of change in the muscarine-like receptors is presumptive evidence of the selective action of microwaves on cholinergic structures.

A very important aspect of the study of the mechanism of action of low-intensity microwaves is the identification of those parts of the nervous system which are most intimately concerned.

Interesting results from this standpoint were obtained by Kitsov-skaya (1968a), who used drugs which induce convulsions in rats and which act on the CNS at different points (camphor, nikethamide, strychnine, nicotine, etc.). She showed that the motor cortex and the basal ganglia, certain structures of the mesencephalon and diencephalon, and the segmental system which controls the transmission of impulses from efferent pathways to the motor units of the spinal cord are sensitive to irradiation. To this conclusion must be added the inhibitory action on nicotine-like cholinergic receptors already mentioned above.

It must be emphasized that the nervous system varies in its degree of sensitivity to microwave irradiation. Its response is most marked to millimeter radiation (as exemplified by the response of higher nervous activity of animals). However, the peripheral nervous system and, in particular, the receptors of the skin, are highly sensitive to millimeter irradiation, even to a single dose.

The functional disturbances develop and attain their definitive state gradually.

Depending on the physical parameters (wavelength and intensity of irradiation), on the duration of exposure, and on the initial functional state of the body, the course of the process may vary, having one or two phases; usually there are two phases, with initial stimulation and subsequent depression of the functions. Investigations have shown that morphological changes resulting from exposure to radio waves of different frequencies and of nonthermogenic intensity also develop gradually.

The morphological changes following exposure to radio waves of low intensity are examined in detail below.

Morphological Changes Following Prolonged and Repeated Low-Intensity Microwave Irradiation

Morphological Changes Following Prolonged and
Repeated Irradiation with Low-Intensity Centimeter Waves

Morphological changes in the viscera and nervous system
were studied in 74 albino rats exposed repeatedly for long periods
to pulsed and continuous 10-cm waves and pulsed 3-cm waves of
low intensity, depending on differences in the duration of irradiation.

Group 1. To analyze the initial disturbances resulting from
the action of centimeter waves, it is necessary to examine in rather
more detail the chronic effects of 10-cm waves of very low intensity on the animal organism. Such a study is rendered all the more
important because these intensities may be encountered in industry.

Repeated exposure (35-40 sessions, each lasting 30 min) of
albino rats to low-intensity 10-cm pulsed or continuous waves was
studied. No signs of hyperthermia were observed. There were
no external manifestations of the action of the centimeter waves.
The animals appeared normal and continued to gain weight equally
with the controls; they were clinically healthy.

The rats were sacrificed at various times after the end of irradiation: one batch immediately after irradiation, a second batch one
week later, and a third batch 3 weeks after the end of irradiation.

No vascular disorders were found in animals sacrificed immediately after the last irradiation. Cloudy swelling of the cytoplasm was found in individual cortical and hypothalamic neurons, with occasionally the appearance of solitary vacuoles in the cytoplasm (especially of hypothalamic neurons), slight swelling, and uneven staining of single myocardial muscle fibers. Histochemical examination revealed a slight decrease in the ribonucleoprotein content in the skin and in several visceral organs normally rich in RNP (neurons, glandular epithelium of the gastrointestinal tract). The most marked decrease in RNP content was found in the epidermis and its derivatives in the surface layers of the skin. Individual animals showed swelling of the cytoplasm and slight cloudy swelling of individual hepatocytes and the epithelium of single convoluted renal tubules.

Not all these changes could be seen 3 weeks after the end of irradiation, i.e., some regression had taken place.

After repeated daily irradiation (34 sessions) for 30 min with 3-cm pulsed waves up to 10 mW/cm^2 in intensity, no external manifestations of the action of the radiation could be found.* In animals sacrificed immediately after the last irradiation the changes were even less marked than after irradiation with 10-cm waves. In animals sacrificed 1 and 3 weeks after the end of irradiation no morphological changes could be seen in the internal organs or brain. Consequently, all the morphological changes mentioned above are reversible.

Hence, in animals irradiated repeatedly with 3- and 10-cm pulsed waves of low intensity (10 mW/cm^2) and whose initial state was good, investigation with the usual morphological methods revealed initial, reversible, and very insignificant degenerative changes, mainly in the nervous system. These changes, according to P. E. Snesarev, are an early response of the nervous system to stimulation. They were very slight, reversible, and compensated, and the animal remained to all intents and purposes healthy.

In animals irradiated repeatedly with 10- and 3-cm waves not exceeding 10 mW/cm^2 in intensity for up to 10 months no ex-

---

*Changes connected with the method of sacrifice (decapitation) were allowed for. All changes described in the experimental animals are relative to a control.

ternal manifestations of their action could be seen. At the same time, it was found that low intensities of 10-cm irradiation, although not giving a thermal effect, nevertheless give rise to certain physiological changes. For example, changes in the CNS expressed as an imbalance between the fundamental nervous processes (Kitsovskaya, 1960), disturbance of conditioned-reflex activity of the animals (Lobanova, 1960), and lowering of the blood pressure (Gordon, 1960, 1964) were found in these animals. The usual morphological methods of investigation, capable of revealing morphological changes of slight severity, failed to reveal any changes accompanying these physiological disorders.

It was therefore necessary to use more precise, elective neurohistological methods to investigate the nervous system, for example, to study changes in synapses and receptors of the CNS, with their very delicate responses to stimulation. It was therefore decided to investigate the higher nervous activity of irradiated animals and to accompany this by a parallel study of synaptic activity in the cerebral cortex after exposure to centimeter waves.

Before describing the results of these investigations, the literature on interneuronal connections in the cerebral cortex must be briefly surveyed.

The morphological organization of interneuronal connections in nerve tissue is very clearly defined. In the human brain, characterized by the high level of development of the association areas, cortical connections achieve an extremely high level of differentiation and complexity (Sarkisov).

Sarkisov (1948) and Polyakov (1955) studied the complex organization of cortical interneuronal connections. They found that three systems (efferent and afferent neurons and interneurons) interact and distribute the flow of nervous impulses over the cerebral cortex and constitute the material basis of the reflex arc. Transmission of the nervous impulse from one neuron to another can take place only through terminal branches of the axon of one neuron to the dendrites or bodies of the other neuron.

Synapses joining neurons and specialized for the reception of impulses or their transmission to other neurons have been studied by Dolgo-Saburov (1956), Polyakov, Sarkisov, and Lavrent'ev. Other investigations (Snesarev, Lavrent'ev, Sarkisov, Polyakov)

have shown that there are two types of interneuronal synapses:
axo-somatic, or direct, terminal connections in which the terminal
branches of the axon of one neuron wind around the body of another
neuron and form synaptic contacts, "boutons," knobs, and rings
(Fig. 15) on it, and axo-dendritic synapses, "en passant," or col-
lateral synapses, in which very fine branches of the axon make
contact with branches of the dendrites. Contact takes place through
very small spines carried by the dendrites (Fig. 16).

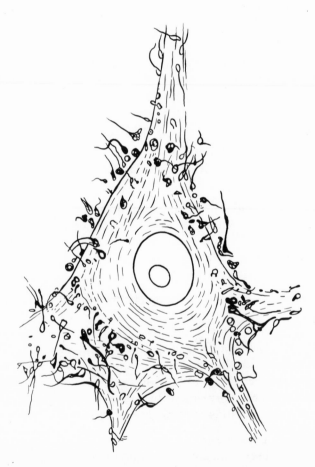

Fig. 15. Axo-somatic synapses consisting of terminal boutons
on body of nerve cell (after Shabadash).

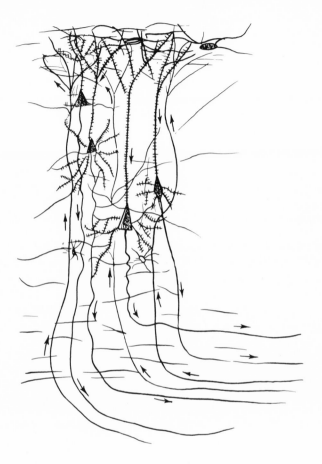

Fig. 16.   Diagram of axo-dendritic synapses in the cerebral cortex
(after Cajal).

The scheme of interneuronal connections in the cortex as
described by Polyakov is as follows. Axons arriving in the cortex
from lower levels of the nervous system branch in the deep layers
and form direct connections between one neuron and another, or
branches of axons in the phylogenetically young, association layers
near the surface of the cortex come into contact with large numbers
of neuronal dendrites in different layers of the cortex, for in whatever layer the efferent neuron lies, it most frequently sends its
apical dendrite into the upper layers of the cortex for association

purposes (Fig. 17). Connections of this type constitute a delicate mechanism for controlling and modifying the functional state of many neurons depending on changes in the functional state of any one of them.

In the human cortex, because of the high development of the association connections, axo-dendritic, indirect synapses are of the utmost importance.

In the modern view (Sarkisov, Polyakov) spines on the dendrites of nerve cells, as cortical receptor systems, undergo changes before the presynaptic axonal branches and their systems of synapses and before the bodies of the nerve cells are correspondingly affected.

An investigation was accordingly carried out in order to study the initial morphological changes in cortical interneuronal connections after prolonged exposure to 10-cm waves of low intensity, to identify the stages of gradual development of changes in the cortical interneuronal connections depending on the intensity of irradiation and to correlate these with changes in conditioned reflexes, and also to study the reversibility of these changes.

Pieces of cortex taken from the motor and sensory areas were impregnated with silver by Golgi's method (some sections were stained by the Golgi-Bubenet method).

As the control, the structure of the interneuronal connections was studied in the cortex of 10 unirradiated healthy albino rats, killed by decapitation.

Examination under high power clearly shows that the apical and basal dendrites of a pyramidal neuron are abundantly supplied with small spines (Fig. 18a). Spines are particularly clearly visible when examined with an immersion objective: they consist of pear-shaped projections of cytoplasm, lying perpendicularly to the long axis of the dendrite (Fig. 18b). Often they appear like small "boutons" on thin pedicles (Fig. 18c).

The largest number of spines was found on the apical dendrites of pyramidal and spindle cells, and on dendrites running from various layers of the cortex into the surface layers for association purposes, and branching there. They were fewer in number on the basal dendrites, and totally absent on the bodies of the nerve cells.

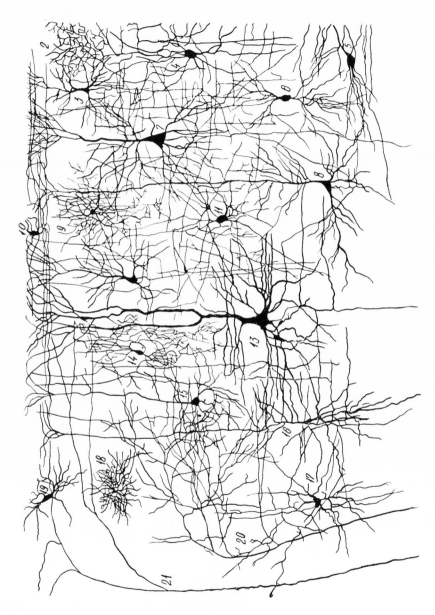

Fig. 17. Polyakov's scheme of interneuronal connections in the cerebral cortex.

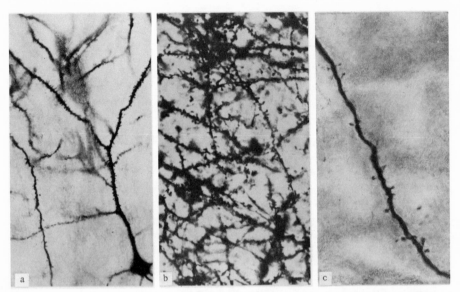

Fig. 18. Comparative characteristics of abnormal and normal axo-dendritic interneuronal synapses (see also Fig. 19). a) Cortical etterent neurons of control rat. Spines clearly visible on apical dendrite and its branches. Golgi, 320×; b) Plexus of apical dendrites in upper layers of cortex. Spines on dendrites clearly visible; they appear as pear-shaped projections of cytoplasm. Golgi, 480×; c) Apical dendrite of pyramidal (efferent) cortical neuron of control rat. Spines clearly visible on dendrite; they appear as "boutons" on very thin pedicles. Golgi-Bubenet, 650×.

Interneuronal axo-dendritic synapses in the cortex were then investigated in a second group of animals after exposure to 10-cm pulsed and continuous waves of between 4 and 10 mW/cm^2 intensity (35-40 sessions of irradiation, each 30 min in duration). The animals were sacrificed by decapitation immediately after the last irradiation. Conditioned reflexes were disturbed at this time. The animals (investigated by E. A. Lobanova) showed weakening of excitation, disturbance of differentiation, and, later, a paradoxical response and limiting inhibition. Examination of sections through the cortex showed that the spines on the end of the dendrites were deformed (they were thicker and shorter) and, sometimes, fragmented; the number of spines was considerably reduced.

When the number of sessions of irradiation was increased the spines disappeared completely and beading and spherical swellings appeared on the dendrite. The apical dendrites running into the upper association layers of the cortex were particularly severely affected. The process began at the end of the dendrites and diminished in severity toward the cell body (Fig. 19). Whereas bead-like swellings can be seen at the end of the apical dendrite, nearer to the cell body the dendrite has smooth outlines and is covered with spines. With a further increase in the number of sessions of irradiation (accompanied by total disappearance of conditioned reflexes) the deformation of the dendrites also spread into the deeper layers of the cortex toward the cell body (Fig. 27a).

Comparison of the morphological changes in the nervous system of animals exposed to pulsed and continuous 10-cm waves showed that the changes were more marked and more distinct after exposure to pulsed waves.

The changes were distinctly focal in character, and side by side with pathological neurons there were always others with a

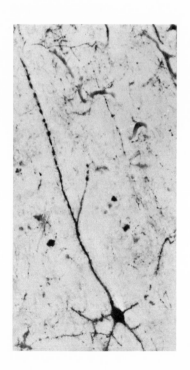

Fig. 19. Comparative characteristics of abnormal and normal axodendritic interneuronal synapses (see also Fig. 18): beading deformation of apical dendrite of cortical efferent neurons of a rat after 2 sessions of irradiation with centimeter waves of low intensity. Golgi, 360×.

normal configuration of the dendrites. In brain tissue stained by Nissl's method the initial changes were found as cloudy swelling of the cytoplasm of individual neurons which, according to P. E. Snesarev, is an early, reversible response of nerve cells to various forms of irritation.

No significant changes except swelling of the cytoplasm of individual fibers in the myocardium, solitary hepatocytes, and epithelial cells of the convoluted renal tubules were found in the viscera of these animals.

All the morphological changes described above in the nervous system corresponded completely with the physiological changes detected on clinical examination as disturbances of conditioned-reflex activity.

In animals sacrificed 3-4 weeks after the end of irradiation, after complete recovery of conditioned reflexes no changes were found in the nervous system. All dendrites had smooth outlines and were covered with numerous spines.

The changes described are functional and reversible and disappear immediately after the end of irradiation side by side with recovery of the animals' conditioned-reflex activity.

The changes described above in axo-dendritic interneuronal synapses in the cortex are not specific for exposure to 10-cm waves; similar changes in these synapses have also been described by Tolgskaya (1954) in animals exposed to various harmful chemicals (arsenic, lead, aniline). They are a manifestation of the fine response of the nerve cells, which may disappear after the action of the harmful agent is terminated, or, conversely, if its action is prolonged, they may be followed by irreversible degenerative pathological changes.

In some rats exposed to the chronic effects of 10-cm waves of low intensity (not exceeding 10 mW/cm^2) axo-somatic as well as axo-dendritic synapses were investigated in the cortex. The former are less conspicuous and are more highly developed in the deep layers of the cortex. The stages of the changes in the axo-somatic loops are illustrated in Gibbs' scheme (Fig. 20).

In the control animals (sections stained by Cajal's method) axo-somatic synapses are very clearly revealed on the motor neurons

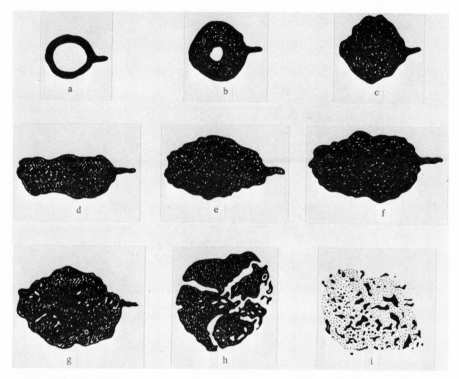

Fig. 20. Scheme showing successive stages of degenerative changes in "boutons terminaux" of the pericellular synaptic system at various times (after Gibbs): a) normal boutons; b) after 24 h; c) after 48 h; d) after 72 h; e) after 96 h; f, g, h) after 120 h; i) after 120 h (granular degeneration).

of the anterior horns of the spinal cord and they consist of axon endings of the ring or "bouton" type on the body of the nerve cells (Fig. 21a).

In the irradiated animals, on the motor neurons of the deep layers of the cortex or hypothalamic neurons these rings and boutons are thickened, their argyrophilia is increased, and the interior of the rings is filled so that they are converted into large "clubs" which are displaced from the bodies of the nerve cells (Figs. 21 and 28), i.e., asynapsia of the neurons occurs.

Consequently, axo-somatic interneuronal synapses, like axo-dendritic synapses, in the brain are extremely sensitive and soon begin to undergo changes during irradiation (before the neurons and cells of the viscera).

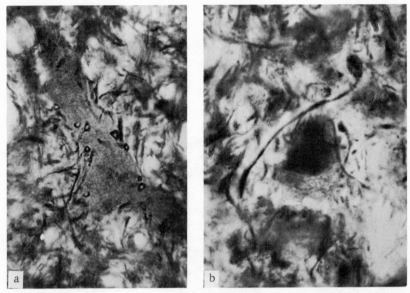

Fig. 21. Comparison of normal and pathological axo-somatic synapses in the anterior horns of the spinal cord. Cajal; 600×: a) numerous terminal loops on body
and dendrites of a motor neuron in the anterior horns of the spinal cord of a control
rabbit; b) club-like swellings and increased argyrophilia of synaptic vesicles and their
detachment from body of the nerve cell in the hypothalamus after irradiation with
low-intensity centimeter waves.

The pathological process in the axo-somatic synapses is reversible, and 1 month after the end of irradiation no sign of these
changes can be found.

Evidently in response to stimulation by 10-cm waves of low
intensity functional reversible changes develop in the synaptic structures of the brain. These changes in the nerve cells, if irradiation
is prolonged, may be converted into irreversible, degenerative
pathological changes.

Besides changes in the brain synapses, morphological changes
were also studied in other fine structures of the nervous system
after exposure to 10-cm waves of low intensity (changes in the sensory nerve fibers of the skin and viscera).

As already mentioned, changes in the sensory nerve fibers
of the cutaneous receptive fields are particularly interesting be-

cause the skin is the first barrier in the way of these radio waves. Because of the very large number of afferent nerve endings which it contains the skin is a powerful receptive field. Waves of the centimeter band are partly absorbed by the skin and partly penetrate into deeper tissues. Changes in the sensory nerve fibers of receptive fields of the viscera are equally interesting. According to published observations, sensory fibers of the viscera respond briskly even to minimal harmful factors.

It was therefore of the greatest importance to study afferent sensory nerve fibers which are so numerous in the tissues of the body and whose coordinated activity helps to maintain the constancy of the internal milieu of the organism. Investigation of sensory nerve fibers in the various receptive fields is an important part of the study of the mechanism of action of microwaves.

Thirty animals were exposed to repeated irradiation by centimeter waves of low intensity (not exceeding 10 mW/cm^2) for 1 h daily and for 100-200 sessions. Changes characterized as irritation phenomena were found in the sensory nerve fibers of the viscera and, in particular, of the skin. They consisted of increased argyrophilia, the appearance of swellings, thickenings, and pools of axoplasm, and marked tortuosity of the nerve fibers. In this group of animals, side by side with pathological nerve fibers there were always many which were unchanged, evidence of the considerable powers of compensation of the peripheral nervous system. The most severe changes were found in the sensory nerve fibers of the skin (Figs. 22 and 29c). Changes in sensory nerve fibrils in the receptive fields of the viscera were equally ill-defined and consisted of increased argyrophilia and the appearance of irregular bead-like thickenings along the course of the fiber (Fig. 30b).

Changes in the nerve cells of the sensory spinal ganglia, nerve cells of the thalamus and hypothalamus, cortical cells, and neurons of the autonomic ganglia (solar plexus, ganglion nodosum of the vagus nerve) also were studied. Swelling of the cytoplasm and tigrolysis in the center of the cell, with ectopia of the nuclei, were observed in the nerve cells of the sensory spinal ganglia. Individual cells showed signs of karyocytolysis and death of the neurons (Fig. 31b). In the hypothalamus the cytoplasm of the neurons was swollen and contained single vacuoles. The neurons of the autonomic ganglia were almost unchanged.

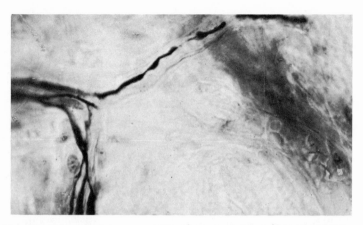

Fig. 22. Skin. Severe argyrophilia of a sensory nerve fiber containing
bead-like swellings and pools of axoplasm. Prolonged irradiation by centimeter waves. Bielschowsky—Gros, 460×.

Consequently, after prolonged and repeated irradiation with
low-intensity centimeter waves, with no elevation of the body temperature and when the animal's condition remained satisfactory,
changes were nevertheless found in the sensory nerve fibers of
the skin and viscera, in the form of irritation phenomena. These
findings concur with the view in the literature that the receptor
system as a whole and, in particular, its preterminal portions are
highly sensitive (Dolgo-Saburov, Pervushin).

This description of the changes in the sensory nerves of the
visceral and cutaneous receptive fields after exposure to low-
intensity 10-cm waves agrees with the writer's previous investigations, which demonstrated changes in the axo-dendritic and axo-
somatic synapses of the brain following exposure to centimeter
waves of the same intensity, giving rise to no integral thermal
effect.

The changes developing in the body in response to irradiation with centimeter waves thus not only depend on the direct action of the centimeter waves themselves on the various tissues and
organs, but also on irritation of the receptor structures of the various reflexogenic zones.

The changes in the sensory nerve fibers of particular receptive fields, giving rise to reflex influences on the central nervous

system and, consequently, on the functional state of the circulatory and respiratory systems, together with changes in the hypothalamic region, could help to explain the fall in blood pressure and brady- cardia observed both clinically and experimentally during the ac- tion of low-intensity microwaves in the absence of any direct ther- mal effect.

Since in these experiments with chronic exposure to irradia- tion of low intensities early changes were found in the hypothalamic neurons it was decided to investigate the hypothalamic neuro- secretory function, more especially because clinicians and physiol- ogists have repeatedly found evidence of the important role played by the diencephalon and hypothalamus in responses to the action of low-intensity microwaves.

A characteristic feature of the response of the body to elec- tromagnetic radio waves is its predominantly vagotonic direction. Clinical and physiological investigations on man (Ginzburg and Sadchikova, 1964; Drogichina et al., 1962) have shown that persons working with superhigh-frequency generators may develop autonomic or vascular disturbances in the mechanism of which an important role is played by the hypothalamus.

There is also experimental evidence of the important role of the diencephalo-hypothalamic region in responses to microwave action.

Evidence of changes in the regulating activity of the hypo- thalamus during exposure to radio waves is also given by the changes observed in the blood pressure of the irradiated animals. These changes were in two directions: in the first period of irradiation by low intensities the blood pressure was raised, but during sub- sequent irradiation it was persistently lowered.

It has recently been shown that the cerebral cortex regulates the various functions of the body, including its endocrine functions, through the pituitary gland.

The hypothalamus participates in: 1) activity of the cardiovas- cular system; 2) thermoregulation; 3) regulation of water, mineral, protein, carbohydrate, and lipid metabolism; 4) regulation of per- meability of blood vessels and membranes; 5) regulation of the functions of endocrine glands; 6) the autonomic basis for somatic functions; 7) regulation of the functions of the gastrointestinal tract and leukopoiesis; 8) regulation of sleep and waking; 9) regulation of the constancy of the internal milieu of the organism; and 10) adaptive behavior, based on connections between the cortex and hypothalamus (cortico-subcortical relationships). Through the hypothalamus the central nervous system thus exerts both nervous and neurohumoral control over functions maintaining the dynamic constancy of the internal milieu of the body and responsible for non-specific internal and external adaptation of the organism to the environment.

The neurohypophysis is formed by the posterior lobe of the pituitary gland and partly by its infundibulum, while functionally it is connected with the anterior hypothalamic (supraoptic and para-ventricular) nuclei.

Axons and dendrites of the nerve cells of these nuclei participate in the structure of the posterior lobe of the pituitary gland. It has been shown in the last 2 decades that neurosecretion is formed in the neurons of the supraoptic and paraventricular nuclei and is transported via the axons of neurons (mainly the hypo-thalamo-hypophyseal tract) into the posterior lobe of the pituitary, where it is stored.

Movement of secretion along axons of nerve cells has been demonstrated histologically. Gomori-positive thickenings and swellings are clearly visible on axons, and at the ends of the axons these swellings assume the form of large club-shaped structures (Herring's bodies), which are particularly conspicuous in the posterior pituitary (Polenov, 1964), where the secretion accumulates around the vessels. Most workers are inclined to believe that the neurohypophysis is merely a reservoir where neurosecretion from the hypothalamus accumulates.

The opinion is held (Polenov, 1964; Voitkevich, 1969) that the secretions of the hypothalamic neurons, like any internal secretion, can enter the blood stream directly (hemocrinia), and this is particularly likely because the anterior hypothalamus has an extremely rich blood supply. Many workers have described the special arrangement of the numerous capillaries in the anterior hypothalamus: the capillaries appear to surround every nerve cell; often the capillaries do not contain glial membranes.

Neurosecretion can also enter the ventricles of the brain directly (hydrocephalocrinia).

Investigations by Soviet and other workers have demonstrated the secretory function of neurons of the anterior hypothalamus both histologically and histochemically. The structural features distinguishing cells of the anterior hypothalamic nuclei have been described: the characteristic arrangement of the tigroid substance (at the periphery of the cell), the eccentric situation of the cell nuclei, and the presence of special Gomori-positive granules and vacuoles in the cytoplasm around the nucleus.

The vacuoles are optically empty or contain oxyphilic colloid. Vacuolation of the anterior hypothalamic neurons was observed by Tarakanov and Maiorova (1957) after injection of hypertonic sodium chloride solution and after x-ray irradiation.

According to Gerber (1967) vacuolation of the hypothalamic neurons is evidence of their intensive activity. The vacuoles may be numerous; sometimes they merge into one large vacuole. The vacuoles burst and expel their secretion; drops of colloid lie extracellularly. In this case the cell has ragged, irregular outlines. This expulsion of large masses of colloid (lumps of cytoplasm) is regarded by some workers as holocrinia (Polenov, 1964). Mosinger (1950) considers that it may be physiological melting of the cell; this is followed by repair. Guillemin (1955, 1961) attributes vacuolation to overproduction of colloid and its expulsion outside the cell. Maiorova describes the complete cycle of secretion of the hypothalamic neurons from the beginning of accumulation to discharge, followed by a process of cell repair. She considers (Maiorova, 1964) that RNP of the cell cytoplasm has an important role in the production of colloid.

Vacuolation of anterior hypothalamic neurons is thus evidently, on the one hand, the highest stage of hypersecretion, while on the other hand it may indicate the onset of degenerative changes in the nerve cells, but in this case the cell nucleus must also be affected (Andersson and Jewell, 1957).

Electron-microscopic investigations (Scharrer and Bergmann, 1949; Mosinger 1950; Voitkevich, 1964) have confirmed the presence of hormonal granules in the cytoplasm of the anterior hypothalamic neurons, along the course of nerve fibers of the hypothalamo-hypophyseal tract, and in the posterior pituitary. Other electron-microscopic studies have shown that granules of neurosecretion increase in volume and size as they move along the hypothalamo-hypophyseal

tract, indicating that synthesis of neurosecretion takes place pro-
gressively as it moves toward the neurohypophysis.

The posterior pituitary contains cells known as pituicytes.
These liberate the secretion from the posterior lobe of the pituitary
gland and deliver it into the blood stream. Pituicytes do not participate in the synthesis of posterior pituitary hormones. Endings
of neurosecretory fibers are in very close proximity to the pituicytes, but there is no neurosecretion in the pituicytes.

The nuclei of the anterior hypothalamus secrete a chemical
substance which is very little different in principle from the hormones secreted by the posterior lobe of the pituitary.

Extract of the pituitary infundibulum contains substances
with an antidiuretic action and with actions on the blood pressure
and smooth muscle of the uterus. These substances are called
antidiuretin, vasopressin, and oxytocin, respectively.

Guillemin and Rosenberg (1957) have shown that, besides
these three hormones, the anterior hypothalamic nuclei also secrete
a substance stimulating the release of ACTH. This factor is called
corticotropin releasing factor (CRF).

Although in the opinion of some investigators the anterior
pituitary (adenohypophysis), which produces gonadotropic, cor-
ticotropic, thyrotropic, and adrenotropic hormones, has no direct
nerve supply, it is nevertheless under hypothalamic control through
the innervation of the portal blood vessels and the penetration of
chemical mediators (hormonal products of the hypothalamus) into
the portal vessels of the adenohypophysis.

The direction of the blood flow along the portal vessels has
now been shown (Zhdanov, 1964) to be definitely from the hypothalamus to the pituitary. This direction explains why the chemical mediators of the hypothalamus can exert a stimulant action
on the anterior pituitary (adenohypophysis), and can exert neuro-
hormonal control over the production of the hormone ACTH (Porter, 1953, 1956; Bogdanovich, 1964). The hormone ACTH liber-
ated by the adenohypophysis induces the secretion of hormones
of the adrenal cortex. The most important of these are the steroid hormones, including the 17-hydroxycorticosteroids and aldo-
sterone.

Zubkova-Mikhailova (1964) found a marked decrease in the production of neurosecretory granules in the nuclei of the anterior hypothalamus and in the posterior lobe of the pituitary after injection of ACTH into the blood stream. Consequently, the neurosecretion has a stimulating action on the production of adenohypophyseal hormones. All these facts suggest that a number of biologically important active substances are produced in the nuclei of the anterior hypothalamus and in the neurohypophysis, and that these substances regulate the activity of the adenohypophysis, and the other endocrine glands by the neurohumoral route (Polenov, 1964; Akmaev, 1960).

As a result of many investigations it has thus been shown that the chemical mediators which reach the adenohypophysis via the blood in the portal vessels can induce its secretory activity. This results in the liberation into the blood stream of ACTH, the principal hormone concerned in the general adaptation response of the organism to endogenous and exogenous demands.

It is now established beyond all doubt that the hypothalamus participates in every physiological and neurochemical process, plays a highly important role in maintaining the constancy of the internal milieu of the body, and is an important brain center controlling adaptation and nutrition (Orbeli).

Polenov (1964) considers that hypothalamic neurosecretory activity is of great importance in adaptation to changing environmental conditions, i.e., that the hypothalamic neurosecretion is important primarily in connection with protective and compensatory responses of the body to constantly changing environmental conditions and to various harmful factors.

According to Polenov (1964) under conditions of stress the neurosecretion is the principal trigger mechanism with a generalized action on the various organs and endocrine glands.

Following the work of Selye on stress and the adaptation syndrome and the investigations of Scharrer and Scharrer (1954b), Bergmann (1954), Mosinger (1950), Aleshin (1964), Voitkevich (1964), Maiorova (1962), and Polenov, Tarakanov, and Maiorova (1957), the importance of the neurosecretory system and the role of the hypothalamus as the trigger mechanism for the hormonal com-

ponent of adaptive responses aimed at the maintenance of homeostasis in the body were realized.

The work of Selye (1950) demonstrated the role of the pitu-
itary-adrenal system in adaptive and defensive responses of the
body to harmful factors.

In Selye's opinion adrenocortical steroid hormones, whose
formation is activated by the ACTH of the adenohypophysis, play
a decisive role in the adaptation syndrome. ACTH formation is
itself regulated by the anterior hypothalamic nuclei. Consequently
the anterior hypothalamus (the supraoptic and paraventricular
nuclei) and neurohypophysis, along with the adenohypophysis and
adrenals, participate in the adaptive mechanisms concerned in the
body's response to harmful factors. Davydovskii (1961, 1962) points
out that the secretory act of the adenohypophysis in response to
stress (to alarm) is probably secondary to the act of neurosecretion
in the hypothalamus. Kurtsin (1963) considers that the pituitary-
adrenal adaptation system can be triggered from the cerebral cortex by a reflex of the following character: the stressor acts on
receptors which send impulses along afferent fibers into the sub-
cortical structures and then into the cortex; from the cortex impulses pass along efferent fibers to the hypothalamus, and from
there by the neurohumoral route to the pituitary gland. The adenohypophysis secretes ACTH which reaches the adrenal by the humoral route, and induces the secretion of corticosteroid hormones
which play the principal role in the adaptation reaction. Since the
same stressors induce active neurosecretion of the hypothalamo-
hypophyseal system and activity of the hypophyseo-adrenal system,
Aleshin (1964), Voitkevich (1964), Polenov (1964), Maiorova (1962),
Tarakanov (1957), and others consider that the production of Gomori-
positive secretion in the hypothalamus (antidiuretic hormone, vasopressin, oxytocin, and CRF) regulates the secretion of ACTH during
stress. Whatever the mechanism of their action, the role of the
neurosecretory system and of the hypothalamus as the trigger mechanism activating the hormonal component of adaptation responses
aimed at maintaining homeostasis in the body have thus been
conclusively proved by numerous authoritative investigations.
The study of the intimate mechanisms whereby hypothalamic neurons exert their regulatory influence is of great general biological
importance. It explains the pathogenesis of many neuroendocrine,
autonomic, and other diseases (Galoyan, 1965).

Many investigators have studied changes in the neurosecretory function during exposure to harmful factors.

Vladimirov (1964) found exhaustion of the neurosecretory system after strong nociceptive stimulation for 10 min. Zhukova (1964) extirpated the superior cervical sympathetic ganglion and observed an increase in the content of secretion in the nerve cells of the anterior hypothalamic nuclei (through blocking of the liberation of the neurosecretion); under these circumstances the blood pressure fell. Consequently, in response to reduced secretion of vasopressin the blood pressure fell. Conversely, in rabbits receiving antithyroid preparations, desympathization was followed by elevation of the blood pressure and a decrease in neurosecretion in the hypothalamus as a result of its discharge into the blood stream in large quantities. Voitkevich (1964) observed a decrease in the content of secretion in the anterior hypothalamic nuclei during dehydration, which he regarded as the result of increased utilization of stored neurosecretory substance in connection with antidiuretic activity. Maiorova found an increase in the content of secretion in the anterior hypothalamic nuclei 2 h after hypophysectomy. Zubkova-Mikhailova (1964) found an increase in the content of secretion in the anterior hypothalamic nuclei and neurohypophysis 3 h after x-ray irradiation. The content of neurosecretion was reduced 24 h after irradiation, and degeneration of the nerve cells began after 6-7 days.

Guillemin (1957) showed that the content of neurosecretion in the anterior hypothalamic nuclei is sharply reduced after injection of histamine into the blood stream. Meanwhile histamine stimulates ACTH formation, and at the same time changes take place in the ascorbic acid content in the adrenals (Galoyan, 1965).

Galoyan (1965) states that after injection of cadmium into the blood stream of animals the formation of neurosecretion is reduced in the cells of the anterior hypothalamus, and this is followed by emptying of the contents of the nerve cells, which then undergo degenerative changes.

According to Aleshin (1965) chlorpromazine lowers the blood pressure while neurosecretion is retained in the hypothalamic neurons, indicating the blocking of its liberation. These findings agree with the observations of Voitkevich (1964), who also observed blocking of the liberation of neurosecretion from the neurohypophysis by large doses of chlorpromazine. Stasis of Gomori-positive secretion is observed under these circumstances in the hypothalamic nuclei.

Hence, the accumulation of granules and droplets of secretion in the hypothalamic neurons may be an indication of its increased synthesis and accumulation, and may also be the result of its deficient outpouring into the blood stream (blocking). No change or a decrease in the content of secretion in the hypothalamic neurons and posterior pituitary indicate increased mobilization of secretion and its discharge into the blood stream, and also the cessation or inadequacy of its synthesis in the hypothalamus. In the latter case degenerative changes affect the neurons of the hypothalamic nuclei.

The results reviewed above can be summarized by saying that in response to acoustic, photic, and electrical stimulation and to whole-body x-ray irradiation in the first stage of stress the content of secretion in the hypothalamus and neurohypophysis is reduced (i.e., the neurohypophysis is emptied); under these conditions the ACTH concentration in the blood rises sharply.

During long-term experiments and on removal of the stimulus in an acute experiment, secretion gradually accumulates. In response to the action of an extremely strong stimulus (stressor) under acute experimental conditions or to inadequacy of the adaptation mechanisms under chronic experimental conditions the neurosecretory neurons undergo exhaustion, vacuolation, and death. Dilated blood vessels and the network of pituicytes can be seen in the posterior lobe of the pituitary gland when deprived of its secretion.

In connection with the facts described above it is of great practical and theoretical interest to study processes taking place in the adaptation system during exposure of the body to toxic substances in low concentrations.

The Soviet literature on industrial toxicology includes many papers on the important role of the nervous and endocrine systems in the mechanism of nonspecific responses (Lazarev, 1963; Spynu, (1959).

Kurlyandskii (1966) showed that in every case of prolonged action of toxic substances in low concentrations on experimental

animals, without exception increased neurosecretion of the anterior
hypothalamic nuclei, the formation of large quantities of neurosecretion in the tissues of the hypothalamus and neurohypophysis,
and the active liberation of this secretion into the blood stream
are observed. These processes coincide in time with increased
activity of hormone secretion in the adenohypophysis, i.e., with
elevation of the blood ACTH level. These changes all indicate a
state of stimulation of the hypothalamo-hypophyseo-adrenal system.

According to Kurlyandskii (1966), besides the disturbances
listed above, changes also take place in other indices: the state
of the descending activating system, arterial pressures, gas ex-
change, and certain aspects of protein metabolism (especially
γ-globulin metabolism).

With all these facts in mind it was decided to investigate
the changes taking place in hypothalamic neurosecretory activity
during prolonged (from 4 to 14 weeks) irradiation of animals (40
albino rats) with 10-cm waves of low intensity (not exceeding 10
mW/cm^2).

As described above, in animals irradiated with such low intensities of radio waves the body temperature did not increase,
the animals' condition remained good, and they increased in weight.
However, 4 weeks after the start of irradiation the blood pressure
began to rise, and after 8 weeks of irradiation it was 13% higher
than the control. This increase was maintained until 12-14 weeks
after irradiation. At the same time the ascorbic acid concentration in the adrenal tissues and spleen was increased. Recalling
that Nikogosyan (1964) and Sangaevskaya (1962) had found an increase
in the 17-ketosteroids in the urine and also of amino acids and non-
protein nitrogen in the blood of animals irradiated for long periods
with 10-cm waves of the same intensity, it could be considered that
the ACTH concentration in the blood of the animals in the present
series of experiments also was increased. All the functional changes
described indicate the onset of compensatory and adaptive responses
in the irradiated animals.

During continued irradiation the blood pressure started to
fall and reached normal figures (corresponding to those in the
control animals) 19-20 weeks after the beginning of irradiation.
If irradiation was continued, the blood pressure fell sharply after

20-26 weeks, and by the 26th week this decrease had become permanent in character. The decrease in pressure amounted to 14-15% of the control value.

Parallel with these functional changes in the animals, the neurosecretion in the anterior hypothalamic nuclei and in the posterior pituitary was investigated histologically and histochemically. The animals were killed by decapitation at different times after irradiation: the first group during the first 8 weeks of irradiation, the second group between 8 and 14 weeks, the third between 14 and 20 weeks, and the fourth between 20 and 26 weeks; the animals of the fifth group (unirradiated) were killed at the same times and acted as the control. Pieces of tissue containing the diencephalon (hypothalamus with the infundibulum) and pituitary were fixed in mercuric chloride with formalin (9:1) and embedded in paraffin wax. Frontal serial sections were stained with aldehyde-fuchsin and methylene blue by Gomori's method in Maiorova's modification. Sections from this same piece of tissue were also stained by Nissl's method.

A study of sections through the paraventricular and supraoptic nuclei in the hypothalamus of the control group showed that the anterior hypothalamic neurons were in different phases of the neurosecretory cycle. A large quantity of Gomori-positive granules could be seen in the cytoplasm of individual neurons. They were most frequently seen very close to the nucleus; the tigroid substance of the cell was displaced toward the periphery. In other cells a phase of discharge of secretion along the axons could be seen. Gomori-positive granules of secretion were clustered together at the periphery of the cell, most frequently near the axon. In individual neurons nearly the whole of the cytoplasm was filled with small Gomori-positive granules of secretion. Sometimes larger Gomori-positive granules and droplets of secretion could be seen in the tissues around the cells and among the fibers of the supraoptic or paraventricular nucleus. Cells of a third group were in a resting state with perinuclear accumulation of small quantities of secretion, and cells of this type in the resting phase were more numerous. When stained by Nissl's method some cells contained tiny vacuoles with granules of secretion. Along the course of the nerve fibers of the hypothalamo-hypophyseal tract, here and there solitary Gomori-positive granules were visible among them. Similar granules were found in small numbers among the pituicyte

fibers in the posterior lobe of the pituitary. Sometimes small
granules in the posterior lobe of the pituitary merged into large
collections (Herring's bodies).

In the animals of the first group, irradiated for under 8 weeks,
a marked increase (compared with control) in secretory activity
of neurons of the paraventricular and supraoptic nuclei of the anterior hypothalamus was observed. Most cells were in the phase
of accumulation or liberation of secretion, and every stage of increased accumulation of secretion in the hypothalamic neurons and
its discharge into the pituitary could be observed in succession.
An accumulation of large numbers of Gomori-positive granules
could be seen in the perinuclear cytoplasm of many nerve cells,
and sometimes the cytoplasm was entirely filled with these granules and the nucleus was displaced toward the periphery (Fig.
23a). In sections stained by Nissl's method, a decrease in the
quantity of tigroid substance and displacement of the nucleus could
be seen clearly in these cells. The nucleus and nucleolus were
swollen and active, with a clearly defined membrane, and many
small vacuoles were clearly visible in the cytoplasm of the cell.
These findings indicated activation of the neurosecretory activity
of the hypothalamic neurons. Neither karyolysis nor death of the
nerve cells was observed.

Sometimes many Gomori-positive secretory granules were
collected near the axon of the nerve cell. Many Gomori-positive
granules were located in the tissues among the nerve fibers of
the paraventricular and supraoptic nuclei along the course of the
axons. Sometimes a subependymal accumulation of Gomori-positive granules could be seen (Fig. 23a). In sections stained by
Nissl's method many neurons contained small vacuoles, as a rule
located peripherally. Some vacuoles were optically empty while
others contained Gomori-positive secretion at the periphery.

An extremely localized accumulation of granules and larger
deposits of secretion could be seen in individual nerve cells inside
the lumen of the large vacuoles. These vacuoles in some cells
were ruptured and the secretion was distributed as large spherical
drops in the tissues surrounding the cell and among the fibers
(Fig. 23b). When stained by Nissl's method these cells had small
vacuoles around the periphery of their body (Fig. 24), and some
when stained with aldehyde-fuchsin and methylene blue gave a

weakly positive Gomori reaction. The nuclei and nucleoli were swollen, with a clearly defined membrane, indicating active functioning of the cells.

The formation of vacuoles in this way is described by Polenov (1964), Levinson (1952), and Bergmann and Hild (1949) as a manifestation of extremely intensive secretory activity of the hypothalamic neurons.

Guillemin (1961) attributes this vacuolation to overproduction of colloid and expulsion of secretion outside the cell (an apocrine type of secretion, with its discharge into the blood and cerebro-

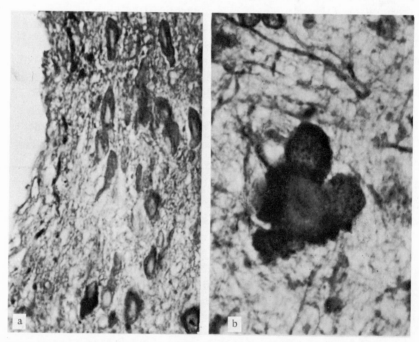

Fig. 23. Neurosecretory activity of hypothalamic neurons during chronic irradiation with centimeter waves. Stained by Maiorova's modification of Gomori's method. a) Rat 3 weeks after irradiation. Accumulation of neurosecretion in nerve cell in paraventricular nucleus of hypothalamus and accumulation of small and larger granules of neurosecretion among the tissues and fibers of the hypothalamus along the course of the axons, 350×; b) Rat 4 weeks after irradiation. Cells of supraoptic nucleus. Cytoplasm of cell and vacuoles at periphery contain granules of secretion. Liberation of secretion into tissues surrounding cell, 830×.

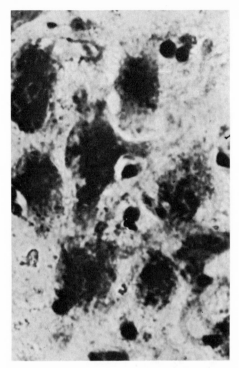

Fig. 24. Swelling of cytoplasm and appearance of single vacuoles at periphery of nerve
cell of supraoptic nucleus of hypothalamus in
a rat 8 weeks after irradiation. Nissl's stain,
675×.

spinal fluid). In individual cells the vacuoles disappeared after expulsion of the secretion and the normal quantity of tigroid substance
was restored. Meanwhile, alongside the cell the expelled secretion
could still be seen as large extracellular spherical droplets of
colloid. The secretory cycle in the cell was beginning to repeat
itself. Very occasionally death of single neurons and evidence of
karyocytolysis with conversion of the neurons into cell ghosts could
be seen. This was the result of excessive secretory activity of the
nerve cell. Much secretion was found inside the neurons also. The
cytoplasm of some neurons was literally packed with granules of
secretion. These cells had lost all their tigroid substance. Many
Gomori-positive granules were found between the fibers of the

hypothalamo-hypophyseal tract, where the granules of secretion appeared like Gomori-positive beads along the axons or as large masses and drops between the fibers of the tract (Fig. 25). As the granules and droplets of secretion moved along the hypo-thalamo-hypophyseal tract their number increased steadily, indicating increased synthesis of secretion along its course toward the neurohypophysis.

Many Gomori-positive granules and larger deposits were seen in the posterior pituitary along the course of the pituicyte fibers, indicating that the secretion is stored in the pituitary gland. The collections of secretion in the pituitary formed Herring's bodies. It was very obvious that some of the larger masses of secretion in the neurohypophysis had broken up into small granules and these lay close to the blood vessels in the perivascular tissue. Sometimes drops of secretion were visible in the vessels.

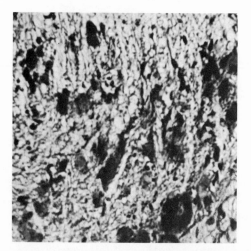

Fig. 25. Neurosecretory activity of hypotha-lamic neurons during prolonged irradiation with centimeter waves of low intensity. Maiorova's modification of Gomori's stain. Rat 8 weeks after irradiation. Numerous granules of secre-tion forming large masses and drops along the course of fibers of the hypothalamo-hypophys-eal tract, 300×.

This indicated an increase in the absorption of secretion and its entry into the blood stream.

Consequently, in this group of animals increased formation and accumulation of neurosecretion and the beginning of its increased liberation into the blood stream were observed.

In the second group of animals, which were sacrificed between the 8th and 14th weeks of irradiation, a completely different picture was seen in the anterior hypothalamic nuclei and pituitary gland.

The nerve cells of the anterior hypothalamus contained a small quantity of Gomori-positive secretion, especially toward the end of the period, i.e., the quantity of secretion in the anterior hypothalamic nerve cells was definitely reduced by comparison with the preceding period. Most neurons were in a resting state. In individual neurons there was no resynthesis of secretion, indicating exhaustion of the nerve cells as a result of their excessive activity in the preceding period. Few Gomori-positive granules and deposits also were found in the neurohypophysis, i.e., there was increased absorption of neurosecretion into the blood. In fact, Gomori-positive granules and drops could actually be seen in the lumen of many vessels in the pituitary gland, and also in the perivascular tissue. Much Gomori-positive secretion was found in the axons of nerve cells in the form of Gomori-positive pools, drops, and granules along the course of the hypothalamo-hypophyseal tract. Granules and drops of Gomori-positive secretion were present around and inside the vessels of the neurohypophysis and even of the hypothalamus, indicating increased absorption of secretion into the blood and cerebrospinal fluid. This coincided with elevation of the blood pressure in the animals of this group and an increase in the ascorbic acid content of their adrenals. Consequently, the reduced content of neurosecretion in the cells of the anterior hypothalamic nuclei and neurohypophysis, together with its increased liberation into the blood stream, accompanied by elevation of the blood pressure and an increase in the ascorbic acid content in the adrenals of animals irradiated with 10-cm waves of low intensity, may be manifestations of an adaptive response to irradiation of this type.

In the animals of the third group, irradiated for 14-20 weeks, marked accumulation of granules of neurosecretion was observed

in the cells of the anterior hypothalamic nuclei, with swelling of
the nuclei and nucleoli, in which the membrane was clearly defined.
Many neurons were in a resting state. The pattern of the neurosecretory cycle was highly reminiscent of that in the control animals. In individual cells of the anterior hypothalamic nuclei
Gomori-positive granules of secretion were observed. Similar
granules were found among the fibers of the hypothalamo-hypophyseal tract, but they were far less numerous than in the first
group. No large deposits or drops could be found among the fibers
of the hypothalamo-hypophyseal tract. Only small Gomori-positive
granules were seen (Fig. 26a). Gomori-positive granules and large
deposits were visible in the posterior pituitary (the neurohypophysis),

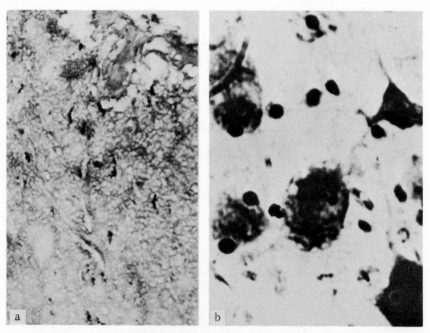

Fig. 26. Neurosecretory activity of hypothalamic neurons after prolonged irradiation
by centimeter waves of low intensity. a) Rat after irradiation for 20 weeks. Small
Gomori-positive granules among hypothalamic nerve fibers. Maiorova's modification
of Gomori's stain, 340×; b) Rat after irradiation for 26 weeks. Marked vacuolation of
some hypothalamic neurons. Loss of nuclear membrane, evidence of karyocytolysis in
individual neurons. Nissl's stain, 680×.

but in smaller quantities than in the previous group. At the same time, small granules of Gomori-positive secretion could be seen in the perivascular tissue of the neurohypophysis. These findings indicated intensive production of secretion and its absorption into the blood stream. Consequently, this group of animals is characterized by the formation (resynthesis) of neurosecretion. Its content in the cells of the hypothalamus and in the neurohypophysis was the same as in the control (unirradiated) animals. Absorption of secretion into the blood stream was observed, because Gomori-positive granules of secretion were found in the tissues around the vessels and in their lumen. The normal content of neurosecretion in the hypothalamus and neurohypophysis correspond to restoration of the normal blood pressure as observed in this group of animals. Here and there cells with tiny vacuoles were observed. There was hardly ever any considerable degree of vacuolation of the nerve cells or evidence of karyocytolysis (with the formation of cell ghosts and death of the nerve cells).

In the animals of the fourth group, sacrificed after irradiation for 20-26 weeks, a completely different picture was observed in the neurohypophysis and in the anterior hypothalamic nuclei. A sharp decrease in the content of neurosecretion was observed in the nerve cells and tracts (axons), and this was accompanied by a sharp decrease in the secretory function of the neurons of the anterior hypothalamic nuclei. Compared with the control group, in this case there was a very marked decrease in the intensity of secretion by the nerve cells. Only occasionally were tiny individual Gomori-positive granules found in the cytoplasm of single cells. Very few Gomori-positive granules were visible in the hypothalamo-hypophyseal tract among the fibers. Many neurons had uneven, or notched, outlines (Fig. 26b). Because of the large number of vacuoles, the nuclei and nucleoli of the neurons were shrunken. Evidence of karyocytolysis was observed. Hardly any secretion was found in the tissues of the posterior lobe of the pituitary (in the neurohypophysis). Only here and there were single tiny Gomori-positive granules found in the tissue around the blood vessels. Neurosecretion was much less abundant than in the control (unirradiated animals). The sharp decrease in neurosecretory activity of the hypothalamo-hypophyseal system was accompanied by a decrease in size of some of the nerve cells, by marked vacuolation of most of the neurons, and by evidence of karyocytolysis of

the cells and total chromatolysis of individual neurons with the
formation of cell ghosts. The nuclei and nucleoli were swollen and
their outlines were indistinct or contracted, indicating death of the
cells. In individual neurons marked vacuolation of the cells and
notching of their outlines were accompanied by shrinking or lysis
of the nucleus and nucleolus (with loss of the nuclear membrane),
indicating degenerative changes in the hypothalamus. In this group
of animals the blood pressure was consistently low.

The morphological findings in the animals of the fourth group,
exposed to prolonged (up to 26 weeks) irradiation with low-intensity 10-cm waves can be summarized by saying that everything
suggests exhaustion of the neurosecretory system as a whole,
with little evidence of the formation and liberation of secretion
and with no secretion present in the depots because it had all been
absorbed previously into the blood stream. No fresh secretion
was being supplied to the neurohypophysis. Clinically in these
animals a consistently low blood pressure was observed.

This description still does not mean that the process in the
hypothalamus is irreversible. Only solitary neurons showed degenerative changes and most of them when stained by Nissl's
method were little affected. Only a sharp decrease in secretory
activity of the anterior hypothalamic neurons was observed, i.e.,
functional changes of a reversible character were present. Some
4-8 weeks after the end of irradiation the neurosecretory activity
was completely restored and corresponded to that observed in the
control animals; the normal blood pressure also was restored.

It can be concluded from the results of this experiment that
three phases depending on the duration of irradiation were observed
in the animals' condition: a phase accompanied by elevation of the
blood pressure, a phase of return to normal blood pressure, and a
phase of consistently lowered blood pressure.

Corresponding to these three phases, three phases of changes
in hypothalamic neurosecretory function could be distinguished.
The first, initial phase is subdivided into two periods: to begin
with increased accumulation of neurosecretion in the cells of the
supraoptic and paraventricular nuclei, followed by its increased
liberation into the blood stream. In the second phase the formation
and liberation of secretion return to normal and its content correspond to that in the control animals. In the third phase the for-

mation of neurosecretion and its liberation into the blood stream
are sharply reduced and neurosecretory activity is exhausted,
with death of individual neurons; this corresponds to the phase of
lowered blood pressure. These findings, together with others
described in the literature and cited above, suggest that in the first
period of the first phase the increase in accumulation of secretion
in response to the action of low intensities of irradiation may be
regarded as a phase of mild irritation with increased formation of
secretion. During more prolonged exposure to the harmful factor,
in the second period of the first phase there is an increased liberation of secretion into the blood stream – the alarm response in-
duced by irradiation (Selye's alarm reaction or stress reaction is
the term applied to mobilization of the organism to adapt it to the
action of the pathogenic factor). This stage of mobilization shows
that the hypothalamus and neurohypophysis, together with the adenohypophysis and adrenals, play an active part in adaptive mechanisms
activated in the response to prolonged irradiation by radio waves.

As a result of the action of these adaptive mechanisms, normal processes are restored in the body (the normal blood pressure
is restored and the content of neurosecretion corresponds to that
in the control animals, but this return to normal is not lasting).

If exposure to irradiation continues still longer, a point is
reached when these compensatory and adaptive mechanisms are
insufficient and break down.

The possibility cannot be ruled out that secretory function
of the hypothalamus is inhibited by the action of the harmful factor
on the cerebral cortex, where inhibition arises and spreads to the
hypothalamus. This can be postulated on the basis of results obtained by Romasenko (1967) and Gerber (1967), who found exhaustion of
the hypothalamic secretory function in patients with schizophrenia
with well-marked cortical inhibition and clinical manifestations of
stupor.

In this period exhaustion of secretory activity of the hypothalamus and neurohypophysis was observed, and activity of the
adenohypophysis and adrenals was reduced. However, this process
is reversible and soon after the end of irradiation all the changes
described above can be reversed and the normal state restored.

The question of changes in the neurosecretory function of
the hypothalamus during prolonged irradiation with low-intensity

radio waves is of considerable interest and calls for further physiological and histochemical investigation of the system as a whole
(including the hypothalamus, the posterior neurohypophysis, the
adenohypophysis, and the adrenals). The investigation now being
described is both functional and morphological in character and
it demonstrates the role of the functional state of the anterior
hypothalamic secretory nuclei, in conjunction with the hypophyseo-
adrenal system, in the adaptive mechanisms arising in response
to prolonged irradiation with low-intensity microwaves in order to
maintain homeostasis in the body.

The results obtained agree with those of investigations by
Gorizontov (1969), who showed that under the influence of stress
factors (electrical stimulation, fixation of animals, irradiation)
reactivity changes in the various periods of the extremal state.
In the initial period, there is what can be called a stage of mobilization (as Selye showed), adapting the organism to the action of the
pathogenic factor. Next follows a stage of increased nonspecific
resistance, and finally there is the stage of exhaustion (Gorizontov).

In animals exposed to even more prolonged irradiation (10-
12 months) by 10-cm waves, in addition to the changes described
above in the fine structures of the hypothalamus and neurohypophysis, slight degenerative changes also are found in the brain, in
the form of swelling of individual cortical cells, and shrinking and
dark staining of other neurons (Fig. 32a). Numerous vacuoles also
were observed in the hypothalamic neurons with evidence of karyocytolysis and the formation of cell ghosts (Fig. 33b). Histochemical
investigation of the skin revealed a decrease in the RNP content
in its surface layers, in the epidermis, and in its derivatives (Fig.
34b). In addition, unevenness of staining was found, and sometimes
homogenization of the myocardial muscle fibers (Fig. 35b).

In individual animals exposed to still longer irradiation (12-
15 months) with 10-cm waves with an intensity of 10 mW/cm^2, in
addition to the reversible degenerative changes in the nervous system
and changes in the myocardium described above there were ill-
defined degenerative changes also in the testes: degeneration of
the spermatogenic epithelium in certain tubules with desquamation
of the spermatogenic epithelium into the lumen of the tubules and
the formation of plugs (Fig. 36b).

In some tubules, besides desquamation of the spermatogenic epithelium, giant cells indicating distorted regeneration were found. However, in the overwhelming majority of tubules in the testis spermatogenesis was normal and the animals were capable of fertilization (as tested by experiments on fertilization of females by irradiated males). Very slight degenerative changes also were found after irradiation for 12-15 months in the hepatocytes and the epithelial cells of the convoluted renal tubules: cloudy swelling of the cytoplasm with the appearance of single vacuoles. Regenerative changes were found in the hepatocytes (the appearance of mitoses and of polynuclear cells), and a proliferative response of the microglia in the brain (Fig. 37b) and of the reticuloendothelial elements in the liver (Fig. 38b) also was present, reflecting adaptive and defensive responses of the body. Despite the prolonged irradiation, clinically the animal remains healthy.

Comparison of the morphological changes found in animals after exposure to pulsed and continuous irradiation with 10-cm waves shows that the changes were more marked in the case of pulsed waves.

Morphological Changes Following Repeated Irradiation with Low-Intensity Millimeter Waves

Animals were exposed frequently (for 10 months) to irradiation with intensities up to 10 mW/cm^2 for 1 h daily.

The animal showed no clinical signs of hyperthermia, but the rectal temperature (as mentioned above) was raised by 0.3°C. The animals tolerated irradiation well. The irradiated animals gained in weight somewhat more slowly than the control animals and showed a slight hypotensive effect.

Morphological examination of this group of animals by the usual methods revealed virtually no degenerative changes in the viscera or nervous system.

However, by the use of delicate elective methods of investigation changes were found in the cortical interneuronal synapses: disappearance of the spines on the apical dendrites of individual cortical neurons with the appearance of beads and irregular thickenings on the dendrites.

Marked changes in the sensory nerve fibrils of the skin, consisting of increased argyrophilia and the appearance of bead-like thickenings and swellings, also were observed. Frequently the fibril was fragmented (Fig. 29a). Axons of larger myelinated cutaneous nerve trunks were affected by the process (Fig. 29b). Changes in the sensory nerve fibrils of the visceral receptive fields were almost completely absent (Fig. 30a). Meanwhile changes were found in the neurons of the spinal sensory ganglia, in the form of swelling of the cytoplasm with tigrolysis in the center and ectopia of the nuclei (Fig. 31a), indicating reversible changes in the ganglionic neurons as a result of reflex stimulation of the cutaneous sensory nerve fibers. This can be postulated because, according to information in the literature, millimeter waves are absorbed in the skin and do not spread deeper into the body tissues.

During continued irradiation changes appeared in the cortical neurons: shrinking of individual groups of neurons with dark staining of their cytoplasm. Swelling of the cytoplasm and the appearance of solitary vacuoles also were observed in certain hypothalamic neurons (Fig. 33a) with an accompanying decrease in the RNP content. Histochemical changes in the skin consisted of a decrease in the RNP content in the surface layers of the skin, the cells of the epidermis, and its derivatives (Fig. 34a).

Consequently, during exposure to low-intensity radio waves changes in the cortical interneuronal synapses, histochemical changes in the skin, and changes in the sensory nerve fibrils of the skin appeared sooner than the usual morphological changes, i.e., they appeared before any changes in the body were detectable by the usual histological methods. Swelling and unevenness of staining of the myocardial muscle fibers were discovered later (Fig. 35a).

The RNP content in the spermatogenic epithelium was slightly reduced. Vacuolation of the cytoplasm of the spermatogenic epithelial cells with pycnosis of their nuclei was found in some of the tubules, most frequently under the capsule of the testis. Occasionally necrosis of the tubules developed, particularly beneath the capsule (Fig. 36a). During prolonged irradiation, tubules with desquamation of the spermatogenic epithelium into the lumen of the tubules and the formation of albuminous deposits were found under the capsule.

Slight cloudy swelling of individual hepatocytes and epithelial cells of the convoluted renal tubules was found later.

Hence, despite the ill-defined degenerative changes in the viscera and nervous system detectable by the usual morphological methods, more delicate methods of investigation revealed more definite changes in the nervous system of the animals of this group (especially in the sensory nerve fibers of the skin and the interneuronal synapses of the cerebral cortex). The changes were most marked in the skin, where histochemical disturbances, namely, a decrease in the RNP content, also were found.

Characteristic morphological changes for the animals of this group are slight proliferation of the microglia in the brain (mainly around the blood vessels; Fig. 37a) and of the reticuloendothelial elements of the liver (Fig. 38a).

Consequently, the slight degenerative changes developing in the nervous system, viscera, and skin in response to prolonged stimulation by low-intensity millimeter waves are accompanied by proliferation of the microglia in the brain and reticuloendothelial elements of the liver. The proliferative changes reflect defensive and adaptive processes in the body.

Comparison of the morphological changes after prolonged exposure to repeated sessions of irradiation with 10-cm and millimeter waves indicates that the degenerative changes in the viscera are more severe in response to the action of the 10-cm waves while the histochemical changes in the skin and changes in the sensory nerve fibrils of the skin are more severe as a result of the action of millimeter waves.

The selective changes in the sensory nerve fibrils of the skin and the histochemical changes in the skin described above are evidently due to the action of waves of this particular wavelength, for millimeter waves are absorbed in the surface layers of the skin and do not penetrate into deeper tissues. It can be postulated that the degenerative and proliferative changes in the viscera and central nervous system during exposure to millimeter waves are brought about by nervous reflex mechanisms. This hypothesis is also confirmed by the irritation phenomena in the neurons of the spinal sensory ganglia.

Morphological Changes Following Repeated Irradiation with Low-Intensity Decimeter Waves

Animals were exposed to prolonged and repeated irradiation with decimeter waves up to 10 mW/cm^2 in intensity for 60 min daily for 10 months (220 sessions). The animals tolerated the irradiation well and there were no signs of hyperthermia. However, changes were observed in their higher nervous activity, and these were particularly marked and appeared early in rats, which are sensitive to acoustic stimulation. The animals also showed a hypotensive effect and their gain in weight was less than that of the control animals.

Investigation of the animals of this group by ordinary morphological methods revealed practically no vascular disorders or degenerative changes in the viscera and nervous system. By the use of delicate elective neurohistological methods changes were found in the complex structures of the nervous system: the cortical interneuronal synapses and sensory nerve fibers of the visceral receptive fields. The changes consisted of disappearance of spines from the dendrites of individual cortical neurons and the appearance of beading and irregular thickenings on the dendrites (Fig. 27b). No changes were found in the sensory nerve fibers of the skin (Fig. 29d), but marked signs of irritation and degenerative changes were observed in the sensory nerve fibers of the receptive (reflexogenic) zones of the viscera (myocardium, aorta, esophagus, intestine, stomach, bladder; Fig. 30c). The nerve fibers showed increased argyrophilia and tortuosity, bead-like thickenings and pools of axoplasm appeared on them, and sometimes the fibers were broken up into fragments. Consequently, the sensory nerve fibers of the skin were not predominantly affected in this case.

During continued irradiation swelling of the cytoplasm of individual cells (with the appearance of vacuoles) of the nervous system was observed in the basal ganglia, and the changes were most severe in the hypothalamus (Fig. 33c).

Histochemical investigation revealed a decrease in the RNP content in the cytoplasm of cells in organs normally rich in RNP (bronchial epithelium, glandular epithelium of the gastrointestinal tract). The RNP content in the skin was not reduced (Fig. 34c). Swelling, irregularity of staining, and homogenization of individual

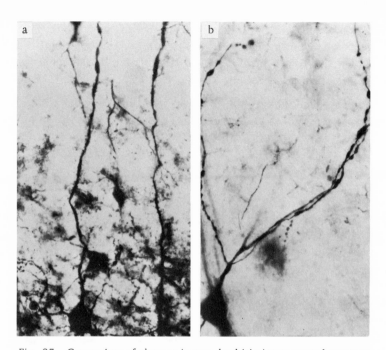

Fig. 27. Comparison of changes in axo-dendritic interneuronal synapses in the cerebral cortex during prolonged irradiation with waves of different lengths and of low intensity. Stained by Golgi's method: a) severe beading deformation of apical dendrites. Prolonged irradiation by centimeter waves, 110×; b) beading deformation of apical dendrites of cortical pyramidal neurons after prolonged irradiation by low-intensity decimeter waves 400×.

muscle fibers were observed in the myocardium (Fig. 35c). After longer irradiation some animals developed degenerative changes in the spermatogenic epithelium of individual tubules of the testes, with desquamation of the epithelium into the lumen of the tubules and the formation of casts (Fig. 36c). Giant cells, a manifestation of distorted regeneration, were found in other tubules. However, only individual tubules were affected and the great majority continued to exhibit normal spermatogenesis. The animals remained capable of fertilization (as tested by fertilization of females by the irradiated males).

A slight degree of cloudy swelling was found in individual hepatocytes and epithelial cells of certain convoluted renal tubules. In the liver there was fatty degeneration of individual hepatocytes with the appearance of minute droplets of fat.

Against the background of the very slight degenerative changes in the brain described above focal and diffuse proliferation of microglial cells was observed, mainly around the blood vessels (Fig. 37c). Microglial processes showed the initial signs of degeneration. Slight hyperplasia of reticuloendothelial elements was observed in the liver, sometimes with the formation of submiliary histocytic nodules (Fig. 38c). The number of perivascular round cells in the lungs was greater than normal. It must be emphasized that besides the evidence of irritation in the fine structures of the nervous system (synapses, sensory nerve fibrils in the various visceral receptive fields) and the gradually increasing degenerative changes in the viscera and testes, there was also a gradual increase in the intensity of proliferation of the microglia in the brain and of the reticuloendothelial cells in the liver.

Comparison of the morphological changes found in animals exposed to the action of low-intensity microwaves of all frequencies clearly shows that irradiation whose intensity is too low to induce a thermogenic effect is nevertheless harmful in its action.

This does not confirm the view, so widely held in the past among Soviet investigators and still maintained to a large extent even at the preset time in the West, that the action of microwaves is entirely thermal.

In the present experiment the attention was concentrated chiefly on the chronic effect of low-intensity microwaves, on the detection of the earliest responses of the body, and the character and severity of these responses in relation to the wave band.

The central nervous system and, in particular, its higher levels are highly sensitive to the action of microwaves, which cause disturbances of conditioned-reflex activity (weakening of excitation and the development of limiting inhibition) accompanied by changes in the structure of axo-dendritic and axo-somatic synapses in the brain. Changes are also found in the sensory nerve fibrils of the skin and viscera.

A decrease in excitability and weakening of inhibition were observed in irradiated rats, animals which are sensitive to acoustic stimulation.

Early responses of the CNS to microwave irradiation were detected by recording brain potentials, and by analysis of the relationship between intensity of irradiation and latent period a curve reflecting the sensitivity of the rabbit CNS to the action of microwaves of different frequencies could be plotted. This curve was found to resemble in its character the Hoorweg−Weiss curve of sensitivity for an electric current and the curve of Tsypin and Grigor'ev (1960) for ionizing radiation.

Lowering of the blood pressure is to a certain extent a specific response to microwave action. The intensity, the time of appearance, and the character of the vascular response depend on the wave band and intensity of irradiation.

Functional changes due to the action of microwaves of different bands are similar in character but differ in intensity, in the time of their appearance, and sometimes in their course, notably in the initial period of long-term exposure. In this period (first phase) increased excitability of the nervous system, hypertension, and increased cholinesterase activity in the blood and organs are often observed. The second phase is characterized by depression of the functional state of the CNS, especially of its higher levels, by a hypotensive effect, by reduced enzyme activity, and by marked morphological changes in the CNS.

The intensity of the response varies with the frequency of the microwaves.

As the authors have shown, the intensity of the response of the CNS to low-intensity microwave irradiation is most frequently reduced with shortening of the wavelength, but at the same time the intensity of the vagotonic reactions is increased.

This general pattern can be connected with the depth of penetration and absorption of different types of microwaves in the tissues. The hypotensive effect, which is most marked in response to irradiation with millimeter waves, can be attributed mainly to the action of the radiation on cutaneous sensory nerve fibers and reflex effects on vascular tone. Meanwhile the response of the nervous system, which is more severely affected by the action of centimeter and decimeter waves, can be attributed mainly to the direct effect of the radiation on the brain structures.

There is no question that the effects of low-intensity microwave irradiation are cumulative. Repeated exposure leads to a gradual increase in severity of the observed changes.

This conclusion is confirmed by the gradual development of increasingly severe disturbances of conditioned-reflex activity of the animals, changes in the responses of animals particularly sensitive to acoustic stimulation, and hemodynamic changes (hypotension, reduced cholinesterase activity in the blood and organs).

Functional changes observed after chronic exposure to low-intensity microwaves are reversible.

The character of generation of the microwave energy, whether it is pulsed or continuous, is not reflected in the ultimate effect of low-intensity microwave irradiation.

Parallel with the functional changes in the nervous system after prolonged exposure to low-intensity microwave irradiation reversible morphological changes in the axo-dendritic and axo-somatic synapses of the brain and changes in sensory nerve fibrils in various cutaneous and visceral receptive fields are found. Coordinated activity of the sensory nerve fibrils and their receptor endings in the receptive fields is a factor maintaining the constancy of the internal milieu of the organism. Later reversible changes are found in the neurosecretory activity of the hypothalamo-hypophyseal system, which is responsible for adaptive reactions of the body to the harmful action of radio waves. The morphological evidence of functional changes in neurosecretory activity of the hypothalamus coincide with clinical manifestations of an initial rise and subsequent fall in the animals' blood pressure. During more prolonged irradiation degenerative changes arise in the myocardium: unevenness of staining and homogenization of individual muscle fibers.

During prolonged irradiation degenerative changes are found in the spermatogenic epithelium of individual tubules in the testes. However, spermatogenesis in most tubules is well marked and the animals are still capable of fertilizing females.

Later, ill-defined degenerative changes develop in the liver and kidneys, where they are accompanied by regenerative changes, and proliferation of the microglia in the brain and of the reticulo-endothelial cells of the liver are manifestations of the animals' defensive and adaptive responses.

Morphological Changes in Animals Following Repeated Low-Intensity Irradiation with Ultrashort Waves

After prolonged (1.5 and 5 months) irradiation with ultra-short waves (USW) with a frequency of 69.7 MHz and of low intensity (150 V/m) the animals appeared well and showed no evidence of hyperthermia.

Microscopic investigation revealed ill-defined changes in the nervous system: increased argyrophilia, and irregular swellings and tortuosity of the sensory nerve fibrils of the skin and viscera (Figs. 29e and 30d). The lesions were not noticeably predominant in the sensory nerve fibrils of the skin or viscera.

Cortical nerve cells were reduced in size and darkly stained (Fig. 32b), and hypothalamic neurons showed vacuolation and, frequently, evidence of karyocytolysis (Fig. 33d), while individual muscle fibers in the myocardium were unevenly stained and homogenized. Some rats showed degenerative changes in the spermatogenic epithelium of individual tubules of the testes, sometimes with the formation of giant cells indicating distorted regeneration (Fig. 36d).

Degenerative changes in the viscera were ill-defined: cloudy swelling and sometimes fatty degeneration of individual groups of hepatocytes and cloudy swelling of the epithelium of some convoluted renal tubules. Together with slight degenerative changes in the viscera, there were proliferative changes in the form of hyperplasia of the microglia in the brain and reticuloendothelial cells in the liver, sometimes with the formation of histiocytic nodules (Fig. 38d), and hyperplasia of perivascular round cells in the lungs, to form cuffs.

If the duration of irradiation was shorter, these changes were less severe.

During prolonged (5 months) and repeated irradiation of animals with pulsed or continuous radio waves with a frequency of 155 MHz and intensity 25-50 V/m and 191 MHz with intensity 10-20 V/m the animals' body temperature was not raised. Clinically, functional disturbances consisting of lowering of the blood pressure and changes in the electrical activity of the brain and conditioned-reflex activity were found.

Morphological investigation revealed shrinking of individual cerebral cortical neurons (Fig. 32c), slight vacuolation of the cytoplasm of cells in the hypothalamus, increased argyrophilia and irregular thickenings of the sensory nerve fibrils of the cutaneous and visceral receptive fields, and very slight degenerative changes in the myocardial muscle fibers.

Degeneration of the spermatogenic epithelium of individual tubules of the testes, with the formation of giant cells by distorted regeneration, was slight in intensity (Fig. 36e), but spermatogenesis was intact in most tubules and the animal retained its fertilizing ability. Slight degenerative changes in the nervous system and viscera (cloudy swelling of the hepatocytes and epithelial cells of the convoluted renal tubules) was accompanied by proliferation of microglia in the brain and of the reticuloendothelial cells in the liver.

All the degenerative and proliferative changes were more marked in animals irradiated with waves in the 191 MHz band and with an intensity of 20 V/m than in those irradiated with waves of 155 MHz and an intensity of 50 V/m.

The morphological changes following irradiation by USW in the 191 and 155 MHz bands were more marked than those observed after irradiation in the 69.7 MHz band. All the changes described above became more severe as the duration of irradiation was increased. However, after irradiation with USW ended, the morphological changes were largely reversed.

After prolonged irradiation of animals with USW in the 191, 155, and 69.7 MHz bands, with intensities not evoking a thermal effect (10-20 and 150 V/m), ill-defined degenerative changes were thus found in the nervous system (mainly in cells of the cortex and hypothalamus, sensory nerve fibrils of the skin and viscera), the muscle fibers of the myocardium, and parenchymatous cells of the testes, liver, and kidneys.

The degenerative changes increase in severity with an increase in the period of irradiation, and after irradiation ends they gradually undergo regression. This corresponds to the clinical evidence of restoration of disturbed functions.

Degenerative changes in the nervous system and viscera are accompanied by proliferation of the microglia in the brain and the reticuloendothelial cells in the liver, manifestations of defensive and adaptive responses.

The morphological changes are most severe after irradiation in the 191 MHz band, less severe after irradiation in the 155 MHz band, and least severe of all after irradiation in the 69.7 MHz band.

Morphological Changes in Animals Following Repeated Irradiation with Low-Intensity Short Waves

During prolonged (5 months) and repeated irradiation with short waves of low intensity (2250 V/m) the animals showed no effects of hyperthermia. Their condition was good at the time of sacrifice. Microscopic investigation revealed ill-defined degenerative changes in the nervous system. Increased argyrophilia and irregular thickenings and pools of axoplasm were found in the sensory nerve fibrils of the skin and viscera (Fig. 30e). No evidence of fragmentation of the nerve fibrils was observed. Damage to the nerve fibrils was not noticeably more severe in the skin or viscera. Shrinking and dark staining of individual groups of neurons (Fig. 32d) was found in the cortex, and the cytoplasm of hypothalamic neurons showed vacuolation, frequently with evidence of karyocytolysis (Fig. 33e). Slight degeneration of the myocardial muscle fibers was expressed as unevenness of staining. After more prolonged irradiation, mild degenerative changes occurred in the spermatogenic epithelium of individual tubules of the testes, sometimes with deposition of albuminous masses in their lumen. However, spermatogenesis was intact in most tubules. After a shorter period of irradiation (1.5 months) all these changes were less severe. Fatty degeneration of individual groups of hepatocytes and cloudy swelling of the epithelium of individual convoluted renal tubules were observed in the viscera and were accompanied by proliferation of reticuloendothelial cells in the liver, sometimes with the formation of histiocytic nodules (Fig. 38e), and by proliferation of perivascular round cells in the lungs.

Consequently, during prolonged and repeated irradiation with short waves of low intensities for periods of up to 5 months the changes observed included shrinking of the cortical cells, vacuolation of the cytoplasm of hypothalamic cells, and irritation phenomena and degenerative changes in the sensory nerve fibers of the cutaneous and visceral receptive fields. Pathological changes in the nervous system corresponded to clinical features observed in the animals (lowering of the blood pressure, reduced sensitivity of the rats to acoustic stimulation, and depression of the brain potentials).

Initial degenerative changes were found in the spermatogenic epithelium of individual tubules of the testes with preservation of spermatogenesis in the great majority of tubules, so that the animals still remained capable of fertilization.

Ill-defined degenerative changes were found in the viscera and were accompanied by proliferation of reticuloendothelial cells in the liver.

Comparison of the action of ultrashort and short waves showed that the pathological changes arising in response to both were similar in direction, although the intensity of all the changes was greater after irradiation with ultrashort waves.

Morphological Changes in Animals Following Repeated Irradiation with Low-Intensity Medium Waves

Morphological changes were studied in animals exposed for 10 months to irradiation by radio waves in the medium wave band (electrical component 180 V/m, magnetic component 50 A/m).

Microscopic investigation revealed a background of very slight vascular disturbances against which moderately severe degenerative changes in the form of disruption of the axo-somatic synapses could be seen in the brain (Fig. 28b). Meanwhile, irritation phenomena were found in the sensory nerve fibrils of the skin and viscera. Sensory fibers of the viscera were predominantly affected, and showed increased argyrophilia and irregular thickening (Fig. 30f). The changes were much less marked in the sensory nerve fibrils of the skin (Fig. 29f). Shrinking of cortical nerve cells (Fig. 32e) and tortuosity of their apical dendrites were found, while in the hypothalamus the cytoplasm of the nerve cells was vacuolated and evidence of karyocytolysis could be seen in individual neurons (Fig. 33f).

Initial degenerative changes, in the form of unevenness of staining and homogenization, occurred in the myocardial muscle fibers.

Some animals showed ill-defined degenerative changes in the spermatogenic epithelium of individual tubules of the testes, with the appearance of giant cells indicating distorted regeneration

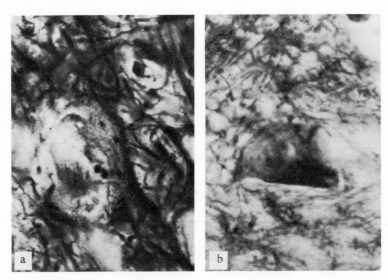

Fig. 28. Comparison of changes in interneuronal synapses in the hypothalamus after prolonged irradiation by low-intensity waves of different frequencies. Cajal's stain, 600×: a) club-shaped thickenings and increased argyrophilia of synaptic boutons and their separation from bodies of nerve cells in
the hypothalamus after prolonged irradiation by centimeter waves of low intensity; b) increased argyrophilia of boutons terminaux and thickening of
synaptic loops with their partial separation from the body of a neuron after
prolonged irradiation by medium waves (magnetic field).

(Fig. 36f). However, spermatogenesis in most tubules was well
marked. The animals remained capable of fertilization during
life as shown by tests involving fertilization of females.

Changes in the viscera consisted of ill-defined cloudy swelling or fatty degeneration of individual hepatocytes and cloudy swelling of the epithelium of individual renal convoluted tubules.

Together with mild degenerative changes in the nervous system and viscera, proliferation of the microglia in the brain and of
the reticuloendothelial cells in the liver, with the formation of
histiocytic nodules in the liver of some animals, was observed.
Comparison of the morphological changes following irradiation by
high-frequency magnetic and electric fields showed more marked
vascular disturbances and degenerative changes in the viscera fol-

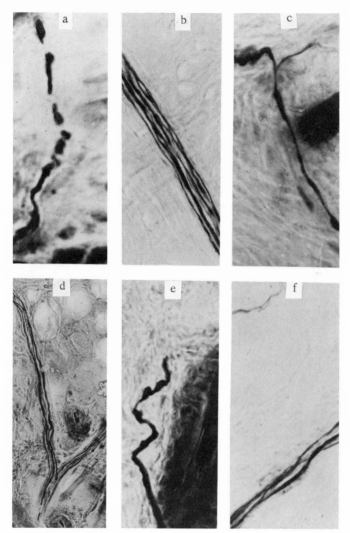

Fig. 29. Comparison of changes in sensory fibers of cutaneous receptive fields after irradiation by low-intensity radio waves of different frequencies. Bielschowsky−Gross stain: a) intense argyrophilia and fragmentation of a cutaneous sensory nerve fiber after prolonged irradiation by low-intensity millimeter waves, 440 ×; b) axons of myelinated nerve fibers in the skin have irregular swellings and thickenings and are strongly argyrophilic. Prolonged irradiation by millimeter waves of low intensity, 330 ×; c) increased argyrophilia, irregular swellings, and tortuosity of a cutaneous nerve fiber after prolonged irradiation with centimeter waves of low intensity, 440 ×; d) unchanged thin and delicate cutaneous sensory fibers after prolonged irradiation by decimeter waves of low intensity, 440 ×; e) increased argyrophilia, irregular thickenings and swellings of a cutaneous nerve fibers after prolonged irradiation by ultrashort waves of low intensity, 440 ×; f) thin cutaneous nerve fibers with slight thickenings in certain places after prolonged irradiation by medium waves (magnetic field), 440 ×.

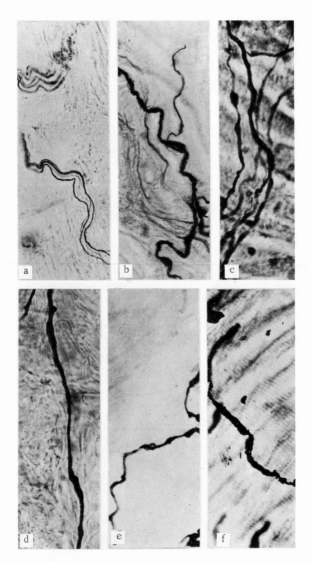

Fig. 30. Comparison of changes in sensory fibers of visceral receptive fields after prolonged irradiation by low-intensity radio waves of different frequencies. Bielschow-sky—Gross stain, 400×; a) almost unchanged sensory fibers of the aorta after prolonged irradiation by millimeter waves of low intensity; b) increased argyrophilia and irregular thickenings of sensory fibers in the esophagus after prolonged irradiation by low-intensity centimeter waves; c) increased argyrophilia, irregular thickenings of sensory fibers in the myocardium after prolonged irradiation by low-intensity decimeter waves; d) intense argyrophilia and irregular thickenings of a myocardial sensory fiber after prolonged irradiation by low-intensity ultrashort waves; e) intense argyrophilia and ir-regular thickenings of a myocardial nerve fiber after prolonged irradiation by low-in-tensity short waves; f) intense argyrophilia and irregular thickenings of a myocardial nerve fiber (near the aorta) after prolonged irradiation by low-intensity medium waves.

lowing irradiation in a high-frequency magnetic field. To sum up, after irradiation of albino rats for 10 months in a high-frequency electric field (1800 V/m) and a high-frequency magnetic field (50 A/m) moderately severe degenerative changes took place in the nervous system (especially in the cells of the cortex and hypothalamus and in the sensory nerve fibrils of the viscera). Degenerative changes were found in the spermatogenic epithelium of the testes and moderately severe vascular disturbances and slight initial degenerative changes were found in the parenchymatous organs.

The degenerative changes in the nervous system and viscera were accompanied by proliferation of reticuloendothelial elements, reflecting defensive and adaptive processes.

Comparison of the morphological changes found after irradiation by low-intensity high-frequency electric and magnetic fields with the changes observed after irradiation by short and ultrashort waves and by microwaves reveals a common direction of the pathological changes after exposure to low intensities of these wave bands, but medium waves give rise to more severe morphological changes than irradiation by short and ultrashort waves and microwaves.

Comparison of Morphological Changes Following Repeated Exposure to Low-Intensity Radio Waves of Different Frequencies (Microwaves; Ultrashort, Short, and Medium Waves)

Investigations of the morphological changes after prolonged exposure to low-intensity radio waves (not inducing a thermal effect) are particularly interesting because it is to these intensities of irradiation that industrial workers are exposed.

To study the action of microwaves, the animals were irradiated repeatedly with microwaves of low intensity (10 mW/cm^2) for 60 min daily for 5-15 months.

Experiments were also carried out in which animals were irradiated daily for 5 months with ultrashort waves with intensities of 150 V/m (69.7 MHz), 50-25 V/m (155 MHz), and 20-10 V/m (191 MHz). When the effects of daily exposure to short waves for 5 months were studied irradiation was given in an intensity of 2250 V/m, while in experiments lasting 10 months the animals were exposed to electrical and magnetic high-frequency fields with intensities of 1800 V/m and 50 A/m. Altogether 243 animals took part in the experiments. It is interesting to compare the physiological and morphological changes in the various organs and systems following exposure to low intensities of radio waves.

119

The animals tolerated irradiation well and no evidence of hyperthermia was observed. However, the irradiated animals gained in weight more slowly than the controls, and certain functional changes were observed.

These were mainly uniform in pattern despite exposure to different frequencies of radio waves, although their severity was identical.

Functional changes can be observed at different levels of activity: subcellular or at the cells, organ, or system level.

Without going into details, it can be said that because of differences in the sensitivity of the various systems to radio waves it is impossible to speak of a single threshold of the biological response to irradiation.

However, it is clear that indices of responses of excitable systems, i.e., neurophysiological data, must be used as the basis for the definition of threshold responses.

Investigations in this direction have begun and will be described in subsequent publications. At this stage, however, it can be provisionally stated that threshold intensities of irradiation for the nervous system in the microwave range are of the order of several microwatts per square centimeter, while in the ultrashort-wave band they are of the order of several volts per meter.

Future investigations are required to obtain more accurate values of the thresholds in two situations:

(1) differential assessment of physiological (especially adaptive) responses;
(2) a differential approach to thresholds of single and prolonged exposure to radio waves.

Morphological examination of groups of animals irradiated with microwaves below 10 mW/cm^2 in intensity and sacrificed after 4-10 months by decapitation, using the ordinary morphological methods, revealed no vascular disturbances or degenerative changes. However, more delicate histological and histochemical investigations using elective methods of staining the nervous system showed initial functional changes affecting primarily the nervous system, corresponding to physiological changes in the nervous system detect-

able clinically, in animals exposed for long periods to low intensities not sufficient to induce a thermal effect. After prolonged irradiation with low intensities changes occurred principally in axo-
dendritic synapses, the delicate receptor structures of the cortex.
The changes consisted of coarsening and sometimes disappearance
of spines of the apical dendrites and the appearance of bead-like
swellings on the dendrites (Fig. 27a,b). These changes coincided
with a disturbance of the animals' conditioned-reflex activity and
were a manifestation of an early, reversible cortical response
which disappeared, accompanied by recovery of the conditioned reflexes, after irradiation had been discontinued.

The bead-like swellings on the apical dendrites of the cortical
pyramidal neurons were equally prominent whatever the wavelength
of the radio waves used.

After more prolonged irradiation disturbances also were
found in the synapses at lower levels of the nervous system (in the
basal ganglia, thalamus, and hypothalamus, where the changes were
found in the axo-somatic synapses) as thickenings and coarsening
of the boutons terminaux and their detachment from the bodies of
the nerve cells (Fig. 28a,b). When irradiation was discontinued
these changes disappeared and the synapses reverted to their normal structure. Marked signs of irritation also were found very
early in the sensory nerve fibrils of the skin (Fig. 29a,b,c,d,e,f) and
viscera, in the form of tortuosity, increased argyrophilia, and irregular swellings of the nerve fibrils (Fig. 30a,b,c,d,e,f). A definite difference was seen in the action of waves of different frequencies, i.e., after exposure to low intensities of irradiation, just as
to high intensities, each wave band gives rise to its own characteristic pathological changes.

After exposure to centimeter and, in particular, to millimeter
waves the most marked changes occurred in the sensory nerve
fibrils of the skin, and changes in the corresponding structures of
the viscera were less marked. After irradiation with decimeter
waves, the sensory nerve fibrils of the skin remained intact but
changes were particularly marked in the sensory nerve fibrils of
the viscera. The action of a high-frequency field was similar. After exposure to ultrashort and short waves, the sensory nerve
fibrils of the skin and viscera were equally affected (compare Figs.
29a,b,c,d,e,f and 30a,b,c,d,e,f).

The sensory nerve fibrils of the viscera were thus affected by waves of nearly all bands except millimeter waves. Sensory nerve fibrils of the skin were affected by all wave bands except decimeter and medium waves.

The disturbances in the sensory nerve fibrils of the skin and viscera were accompanied by reversible morphological changes in neurons of the spinal sensory ganglia, which are the first structures to receive stimuli from the nerve fibrils of the skin and viscera (Fig. 31a,b). The discovery of these changes in neurons of the spinal ganglia after irradiation with millimeter waves confirms the view that the action of these waves is reflex in character, because they are absorbed in the skin. However, by stimulating the sensory nerve fibrils of the skin they give rise to reflex stimulation of neurons in the spinal ganglia.

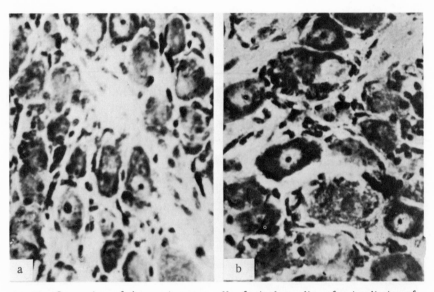

Fig. 31. Comparison of changes in nerve cells of spinal ganglion after irradiation of animals by low-intensity radio waves of different frequencies. Nissl's stain, 530×: a) central tigrolysis and swelling of cytoplasm with ectopia of nucleus after irradiation with millimeter waves; b) swelling and tigrolysis of cytoplasm, evidence of karyocytolysis, and death of individual neurons after irradiation with centimeter waves.

After more prolonged irradiation definite changes were detected in the bodies of the cortical neurons, namely, shrinking and dark staining of individual neurons (Fig. 32a,b,c,d,e). Neurons with swollen cytoplasm containing tiny vacuoles were seen at lower levels in the brain, particularly in the thalamus, hypothalamus, and medulla. Neurons in a state of karyocytolysis also were found (Fig. 33a,b,c,d,e,f). This corresponds to the decrease in ribonucleoprotein content in the swollen nerve cells and, in particular, in neurons containing vacuoles. Changes in the hypothalamic neurons occurred simultaneously with disturbance of the neurosecretory activity of the hypothalamo-hypophyseal system (compare Figs.23a,b; 25; 26). This shows that the hypothalamus and neurohypophysis, together with the adenohypophysis and adrenals, play an active part in the adaptive and compensatory mechanisms. The changes in the hypothalamic neurosecretory function described above were reflected clinically in raised blood pressure. Exhaustion of the neurosecretory activity and a fall of blood pressure then occurred. These phenomena also disappeared after the end of irradiation. After prolonged irradiation at low intensities, histochemical tests revealed a decrease in the RNP content of the skin (Fig. 34a,b,c). Here again, differences were noted following the action of waves of different bands: after irradiation with millimeter waves the decrease in RNP content in the skin was particularly marked, while after irradiation with centimeter waves it was less marked, and after irradiation with decimeter waves the RNP content in the skin was unchanged.

All these findings indicate that the initial functional changes in the fine structures of the nervous system and in the protein metabolism of the cells can be detected by histochemical methods and by elective methods of investigation of the nervous system, whereas no changes are revealed by the ordinary morphological methods.

After even more prolonged irradiation by low-intensity waves of different frequencies changes appeared in the individual muscle fibers of the myocardium (Fig. 35a,b,c) which showed unevenness of staining: some fibers were pale while others were dark and homogenized, but their cross-striation was everywhere intact. These changes were reversible in character. Only occasionally could intensely stained fibrils which had lost their cross-striation

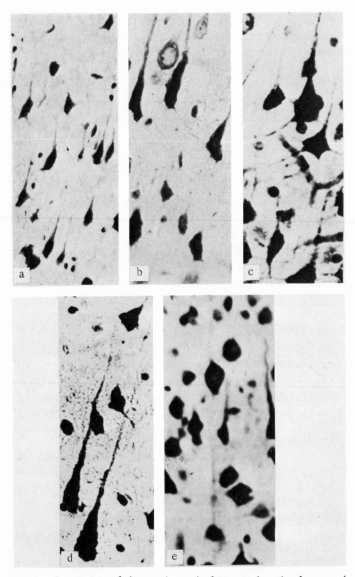

Fig. 32. Comparison of changes in cortical neurons in animals exposed to prolonged low-intensity irradiation with radio waves of different frequencies. Shrinkage and dark staining of cortical neurons. Nissl's stain: a) irradiation with centimeter waves, 230×; b) with ultrashort waves (69.7 MHz), 410×; c) with ultrashort waves (155 MHz), 460×; d) with short waves, 460×; e) with medium waves (magnetic field), 280×.

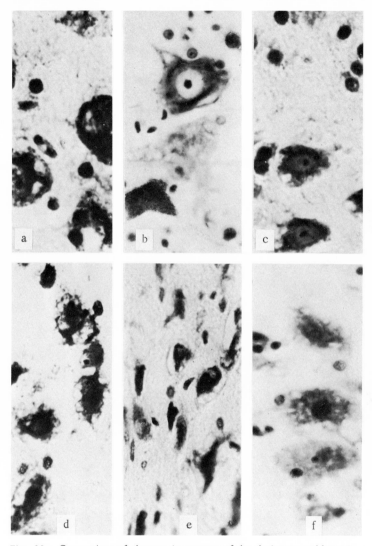

Fig. 33. Comparison of changes in neurons of the thalamus and hypo-thalamus after prolonged irradiation by low-intensity waves of different frequencies. Vacuolation of thalamic and hypothalamic neurons with evidence of karyocytolysis of individual neurons. Nissl's stain: a) ir-radiation with millimeter waves, 690×; b) with centimeter waves, 690×; c) with decimeter waves, 620×; d) with ultrashort waves (69.7 MHz), 620×; e) with short waves, 460×; f) with medium waves (electric field), 690×.

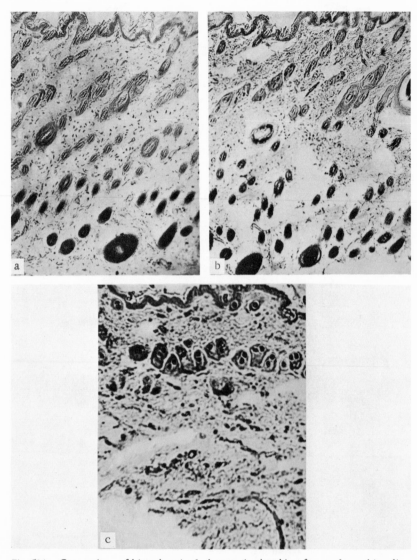

Fig. 34. Comparison of histochemical changes in the skin after prolonged irradiation with low-intensity waves of different frequencies. Brachet's reaction: a) decrease in RNP content in epidermis and its derivatives in the skin after prolonged irradiation with low-intensity millimeter waves 330×; b) decrease in RNP content in epidermis and its derivatives in the skin after prolonged irradiation with low-intensity centimeter waves, 330×; c) normal RNP content in epidermis and its derivatives after prolonged irradiation by low-intensity decimeter waves, 220×.

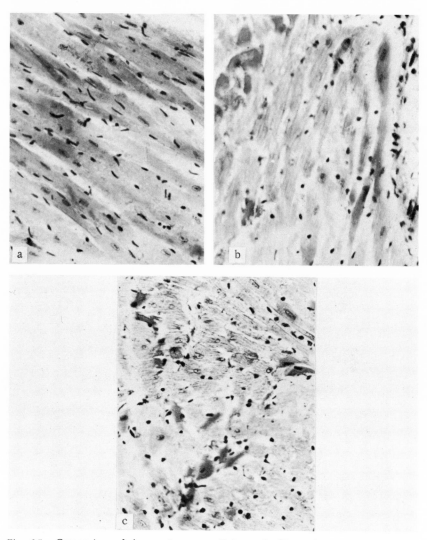

Fig. 35. Comparison of changes in myocardial muscle fibers after prolonged irradiation by low-intensity waves of different frequencies. Hematoxylin-eosin, 330×: a) uneven staining of myocardial muscle fibers after irradiation of animals with low-intensity millimeter waves; b) uneven staining and homogenization of individual myocardial muscle fibers after irradiation of animals with low-intensity centimeter waves; c) uneven staining and homogenization of individual myocardial muscle fibers after irradiation of the animals with low-intensity decimeter waves.

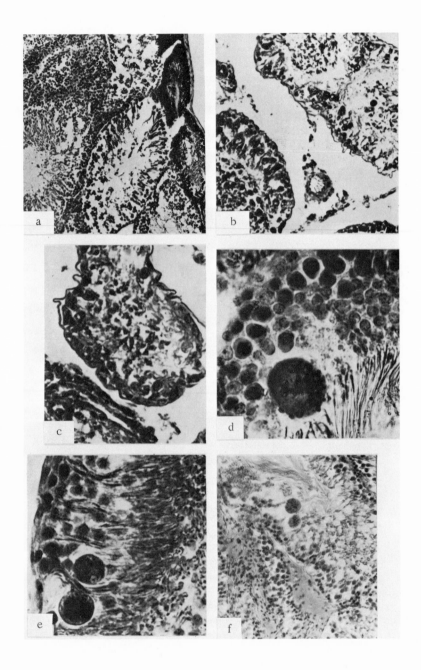

Fig. 36. Comparison of changes in the testes after prolonged irradiation of animals by low-intensity waves of different frequencies. Hematoxylin-eosin. a) Necrosis of two tubules of the testis located beneath the capsule after prolonged irradiation by millimeter waves, 300×. b) Degenerative changes in the spermatogenic epithelium of a tubule of the testis. Desquamation of spermatogenic epithelium into lumen of tubules with the formation of a cast after irradiation with centimeter waves, 350×. c) Degenerative changes in the spermatogenic epithelium with desquamation into lumen of a tubule after irradiation with decimeter waves, 350×. d) Degenerative changes in spermatogenic epithelium with desquamation into lumen of a tubule. Formation of a giant cell reflecting distorted regeneration after irradiation with ultrashort waves, 600×. e) Degenerative changes in spermatogenic epithelium with its desquamation into lumen of a tubule. Appearance of giant cells reflecting distorted regeneration after irradiation with ultrashort waves, 500×. f) Edema of stroma of a testis and desquamation of degenerated epithelium into lumen of a tubule. Formation of giant cells reflecting distorted regeneration after irradiation with medium waves (magnetic field), 400×.

be found. Consequently, the severest changes were found in the nervous system, including neurons, synapses, and sensory nerve endings of the various receptive (reflexogenic) fields.

The structures in second place as regards the severity of the lesions are the myocardial muscle fibers, followed in third place by the testis, in which after very prolonged low-intensity irradiation with waves of all frequencies degenerative changes were found: swelling and degeneration of the spermatogenic epithelium in individual tubules with death of some cells and their desquamation into the lumen of the tubules, sometimes with devastation of the spermatogenic layers and the development of giant, multinuclear cells, indicating distorted regeneration (Fig. 36a,b,c,d,e,f). Waves of all frequencies have roughly the same action on the testis. The changes are slightly more severe after irradiation with decimeter and centimeter waves (in the microwave group), followed, in order of diminishing severity, by ultrashort, short, and medium waves and high-frequency fields. However, only some of the tubules of the testes were affected. In the great majority of tubules spermatogenesis remained intact and the animal was still capable of fertilizing the female, as tests with the irradiated males showed.

After very prolonged irradiation, slight cloudy swelling and vacuolation of the cytoplasm were found in individual hepatocytes

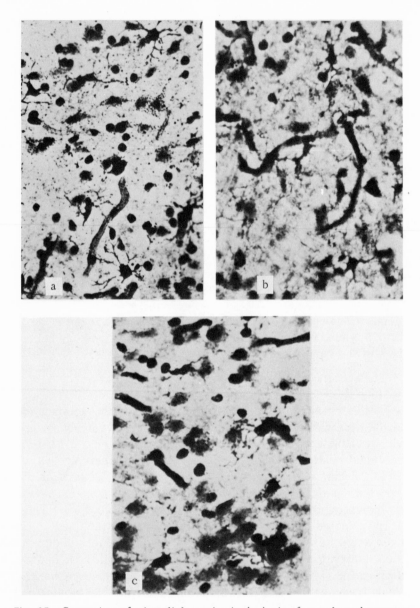

Fig. 37. Comparison of microglial reaction in the brain after prolonged exposure to low-intensity irradiation by waves of different frequencies. Miyagawa–Aleksandrovskaya stain, 330×: a) hyperplasia of microglia in the brain after prolonged exposure to low-intensity irradiation by millimeter waves; b) hyperplasia of microglia in the brain after prolonged exposure to low-intensity irradiation with centimeter waves; c) hyperplasia of microglia in the brain, commencing degeneration of microgliocytes after prolonged irradiation with low-intensity decimeter waves.

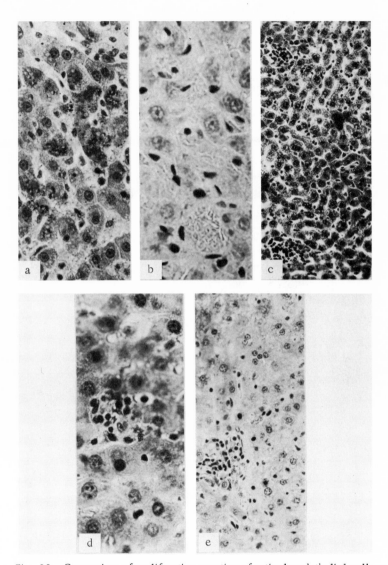

Fig. 38. Comparison of proliferative reaction of reticuloendothelial cells in the liver of animals after prolonged irradiation by low-intensity waves of different frequency. Hematoxylin-eosin: a) irradiation with millimeter waves, 340×; b) irradiation with centimeter waves, 340×; c) irradiation with decimeter waves, 225×; d) irradiation with ultrashort waves, 275×; e) irradiation with short waves, 340×.

and epithelial cells of certain convoluted renal tubules. In some animals (most frequently after exposure to decimeter waves) fatty degeneration of individual groups of hepatocytes, with deposition of fine droplets of fat in the cells, was observed. After prolonged irradiation at low intensities no vascular changes were found. Degenerative changes in the parenchymatous organs were minimal and were accompanied by regeneration (by the appearance of multinuclear cells and mitoses in the liver), and also by a well-marked proliferative reaction of the microglia in the brain, with slight degenerative changes in individual microgliocytes, in the case of exposure to decimeter waves (Fig. 37a,b,c), and by proliferation of the reticuloendothelial cells in the liver, sometimes with the formation of histiocytic nodules (Fig. 38a,b,c,d,e).

Consequently, in response to irradiation at low intensities, besides trivial and mainly reversible changes in the nervous system and parenchymatous organs, a definite proliferative reaction of the reticuloendothelial elements arises. This reaction reflects defensive and adaptive processes in the body in response to low-intensity irradiation.

Conclusion

It can be concluded from the foregoing facts that after irradiation with millimeter waves the most seriously affected structures are the sensory nerve fibrils of the skin, the action being accompanied by histochemical changes in the skin. Irradiation with centimeter waves gives rise to considerable histochemical changes
and also to structural changes in the sensory nerve fibrils of the
skin and viscera and in the interneuronal synapses of the cerebral
cortex. Exposure to decimeter waves and to high-frequency radiation causes damage primarily to the sensory nerve fibrils of the
viscera, unaccompanied by corresponding changes in the sensory
nerve fibrils of the skin; these changes correspond to the more
marked morphological changes in the viscera (in material examined
by the usual morphological methods). After irradiation with ultrashort and short waves of low intensity the sensory nerve fibrils
are equally affected in the skin and viscera.

A likely hypothesis is that millimeter waves are absorbed
in the surface layers of the skin, and that all the degenerative
changes in the brain and viscera are reflex in origin, whereas
decimeter waves, which can penetrate deeper, can affect the viscera and brain directly while leaving the skin intact. Centimeter
waves, which are partly absorbed by the skin, can give rise to
changes in it and also in the deeper tissues.

In response to the action of low-intensity radio waves of different frequencies two phenomena can evidently arise: (a) the wave
can penetrate deeply and exert a direct action on the organs and
tissues (this is particularly marked in the case of decimeter waves),

and (b) irritation of peripheral receptor structures giving rise to reflex effects on the viscera and nervous system (millimeter waves).

During the action of microwaves the animals are in a formed field and they are therefore exposed to a definite flux of electromagnetic energy, while during exposure to ultrashort and short waves and to high-frequency fields the animal is in an unformed electromagnetic field, the intensity of which was indicated above.

The dynamics of evolution of the pathological process during exposure to low-intensity radio waves of different frequencies can be pictured as follows. Although low intensities do not raise the body temperature and produce hyperthermia, in the case of very prolonged exposure they can exert definite effects on the living organism. Electromagnetic waves of different frequencies initially stimulate the sensory nerve fibrils of the cutaneous receptive fields (this applies in particular to millimeter and centimeter waves) or, as they penetrate more deeply, they stimulate the sensory nerve fibrils of visceral receptive fields. It is predominantly the neurons of the corresponding sensory spinal ganglia which respond to this stimulation. The stimulation next passes to the fine structures of the brain (interneuronal synapses of the cerebral cortex, constituting the cortical receptor apparatus), the stimulation in this case being either reflex (irradiation with millimeter waves) or direct, through penetration of the electromagnetic waves into the deeper structures of the body (decimeter and longer waves). Synapses at lower levels of the central nervous system and sensory nerve fibrils of the viscera then become involved in the process. These visceral fibrils constitute an adaptive apparatus which maintains the equilibrium between the internal medium of the body and the external environment (the equilibrium on which the normal existence of the organism is based).

As a result of excessive stimulation of the sensory nerve fibrils of the various visceral receptive fields pathological impulses are sent to the brain, where they induce considerable changes in its nerve cells: shrinking of the cortical cells, swelling and vacuolation of the cytoplasm of the hypothalamic neurons. The neurosecretory function of the hypothalamo-hypophyseal system is disturbed, and this, in turn, disturbs neuroendocrine correlation. This is undoubtedly an important factor in the development of still more marked changes in the nervous system and viscera.

The changes in the fine structure of the cerebral cortex observed in the course of this investigation correspond to clinical manifestations in the form of depression of the conditioned reflexes of the irradiated animals and a decrease in their sensitivity to acoustic stimulation. Changes in the neuroendocrine function of the hypothalamo-hypophyseal system correspond to clinical manifestations reflected by a decrease in the blood pressure.

However, all the changes described above, whether structural or functional, are reversible and disappear soon after the end of irradiation.

All the fine changes described above in the nervous system are found before changes detectable by the usual morphological methods, and they constitute the early response of the nervous system to the action of low-intensity radio waves of different frequencies.

Later in the course of irradiation more marked changes arise in the central nervous system and in the sensory nerve fibrils of the viscera, especially of the myocardium (from this point of view the results agree with those obtained by V. Yu. Pervushin), and they are accompanied by corresponding changes in the myocardial muscle fibers.

During more prolonged irradiation degenerative changes arise in the spermatogenic epithelium of individual tubules of the testes, although spermatogenesis in the great majority of tubules remains intact and the animals are still capable of carrying out fertilization (as tests with the irradiated males showed). Degenerative changes in individual groups of cells in the liver and epithelium of the convoluted renal tubules appear later still.

All the degenerative changes in the parenchymatous organs are slight in degree and are accompanied by a proliferative reaction of the reticuloendothelial cells of the liver and of the microglia in the brain; this reaction is a reflection of protective and adaptive processes.

After prolonged irradiation with low-intensity radio waves, although the animal remains clinically healthy and no detectable thermogenic effect is observed, nevertheless certain reversible and irreversible morphological and physiological changes arise in the body.

For instance, if the effects of radio waves of low intensity but of different frequencies are compared it will be noted that after prolonged and repeated irradiation (lasting up to 10 months) with low-intensity radio waves of the ultrashort, short, and medium bands no significant differences could be found in the severity of the changes in the sensory nerve fibrils of the skin and viscera. However, after irradiation with decimeter and high-frequency waves, the sensory nerve fibers of the cutaneous receptive fields are unaffected although the sensory nerve fibrils of the viscera show pathological changes. After irradiation with millimeter waves, on the other hand, the sensory nerve fibrils of the skin are particularly severely affected, while those of the visceral receptive fields are intact.

After exposure to ultrashort, short, and centimeter waves the sensory nerve fibrils of the viscera are affected equally.

The most severe changes are found in the nervous system and, in particular, in its fine structures: the cortical synapses, axosomatic synapses of the thalamus and hypothalamus, and the sensory nerve fibrils of the cutaneous and visceral receptive fields. Cortical and hypothalamic neurons are particularly severely affected. Neurosecretory function in the hypothalamus is disturbed, and degenerative changes then develop in the hypothalamus, giving rise to vacuolation of its nerve cells; this coincides with a lowering of the animals' blood pressure.

In second place after the nervous system in order of severity of the lesions is the heart muscle.

The third place after exposure to radio waves of all bands (microwaves, ultrashort, short, and medium waves) is occupied by the changes in the testes. After very prolonged irradiation degenerative changes arise in the spermatogenic epithelium of individual tubules although in the great majority of tubules spermatogenesis is unimpaired. This is reflected clinically in the ability of the animals to fertilize the female.

Degenerative changes in the remaining viscera are minimal. They are accompanied by regenerative and proliferative processes, namely, proliferation of microglia in the brain and of reticuloendothelial cells in the liver, and by the formation of perivascular cuffs of round cells in the lungs.

The morphological changes following exposure to radio waves of the whole range of frequencies are basically in the same direction although the intensity of the changes diminishes as the wavelength increases.

In the microwave band the centimeter waves give rise to the most severe changes. Consequently, the most marked changes are found as a result of exposure to superhigh frequencies, followed by ultrashort and short waves, while the least severe effects are observed after exposure to electrical and magnetic high-frequency fields.

Bibliography

Akmaev, I. G., 1960 "The Adenohypophysis, Its Secretory Activity
    and Nervous Regulation," Author's Abstract of Candidate's
    Dissertation, Moscow.
Aleshin, B. V., 1964, in: Neurosecretory Elements and Their Role
    in the Organism [in Russian], Izd. AN SSSR.
Andersson, B. and Jewell, P., 1957, J. Endrocrinol., 15(3):332.
Andersson, B. and Jewell, P. 1958, Acta Anat. (Basel), Vol. 35.
Bach, S., Luzzio, A., and Brownell, A., 1961, in: Biological Effects
    of Microwave Radiation, Plenum Press, New York, p. 117.
Bergmann, W., 1954, Das Zwischenhirn-Hypophysensystem, Berlin.
Bergmann, W., and Hild, W., 1949, Acta Anat. (Basel), 8:264.
Bereznitskaya, A. N., 1968, in: Work Hygiene and Biological Ac-
    tion of Radio Waves. Proceedings of the 3rd All-Union
    Symposium on June 24-28 [in Russian], Moscow, pp. 11 and 13.
Bogdanovich, N. K., 1964a, Arkh. Pat., 26:3.
Bogdanovich, N. K., 1964b, Arkh. Pat., 26:8.
Bovsen, I. E., 1953, Arch. Indust. Hyg. Occup. Med., 7(6):516.
Bykov, K. M., and Kurtsin, I. T., Cortico-Visceral Pathology [in
    Russian], Leningrad (1960).
Chernigovskii, V. N., 1941, "Investigations of the Receptors of
    Certain Internal Organs," Dissertation, Leningrad.
Chernigovskii, V. N., 1959, Vestn. Akad. Med. Nauk SSSR, 4:3.
Cook, H. F., 1952, Brit. J. Appl. Phys., 3:249.
Davydovskii, I. V., 1961, General Human Pathology [in Russian],
    Moscow.
Davydovskii, I. V., 1962, The Problem of Causality (Etiology) in
    Medicine [in Russian], Moscow.

Deichmann, W., et al., 1959, J. Occup. Med., 1:369.

Denier, A., 1933, Arch. d'Electr. Med., 41:273.

Derevyagin, M. P., 1939, Fizioterapiya, 6:55.

Dolgo-Saburov, B. A., 1956, The Neuron Theory—The Basis of Modern Views on the Structure and Function of the Nervous System [in Russian], Leningrad.

Dolina, L. A., 1959, in: Work Hygiene and the Biological Action of Radio Waves [in Russian], Moscow, p. 44.

Drogichina, E. A., et al., 1962, Gig. Truda i Prof. Zabol., 1:28.

Drogichina, E. A., and Sadchikova, M. N., 1964, "The Biological Action of Radio Waves," Transactions of the Institute of Work Hygiene and Occupational Diseases, Academy of Medical Sciences of the USSR [in Russian], No. 2, Moscow, p. 105.

Drogichina, E. A., and Sadchikova, M. N., 1968, in: Work Hygiene and the Biological Action of Radio Waves. Proceedings of the 3rd All-Union Symposium on June 24-28 [in Russian], Moscow, p. 42.

Falin, L. I., 1948, in: Morphology of the Sensory Innervation of the Viscera [in Russian], Izd. AMN SSSR, p. 126.

Franke, V. A., 1960, Collected Scientific Transactions of the Institute of Work Safety of the All-Union Central Committee of Trade Unions [in Russian], No. 3, p. 36.

Fukalova, P. P., 1964, in: The Biological Action of Radio Waves. Transactions of the Institute of Work Hygiene and Occupational Diseases, Academy of Medical Sciences of the USSR [in Russian], Moscow, No. 2, p. 78.

Fukalova, P. P., 1968, in: The Biological Action of Radio Waves. Transactions of the Institute of Work Hygiene and Occupational Diseases, Academy of Medical Sciences of the USSR [in Russian], No. 3, Moscow, p. 101.

Galoyan, A. A., 1965, Some Problems in the Biochemistry of Hypothalamic Regulation [in Russian], Erevan.

Gerber, E. L., 1967, "Neurosecretory Activity in Various Mental Diseases," Author's Abstract of Doctoral Dissertation.

Gillerson, A. V., and Voznaya, A. N., 1939, in: Problems in Experimental Physiotherapy [in Russian], Moscow, p. 149.

Ginzburg, D. A., and Sadchikova, M. N., 1964, in: The Biological Action of Radio Waves. Transactions of the Institute of Work Hygiene and Occupational Diseases, Academy of Medical Sciences of the USSR, No. 2, Moscow, p. 126.

Glezer, A. Ya., 1937, Proceedings of the Leningrad Conference
    on Ultrahigh Frequency Radiation [in Russian], Leningrad, p. 5.
Golysheva, K. P., and Andriyasheva, M. N., 1937, in: Biological
    Action of Ultrahigh-Frequency Radiation [in Russian], Mos-
    cow, p. 309.
Gordon, Z. V., 1960, in: The Biological Action of Superhigh Fre-
    quencies. Proceedings of the Institute of Work Hygiene and
    Occupational Diseases, Academy of Medical Sciences of the
    USSR, No. 1, Moscow, pp. 5-8, 22-25, 65-69.
Gordon, Z. V., 1964, in: Biological Action of Radio Waves. Tran-
    sactions of the Institute of Work Hygiene and Occupational
    Diseases, Academy of Medical Sciences of the USSR, No. 2,
    Moscow, pp. 3-9, 57-60.
Gordon, Z. V., 1966, in: Problems in Work Hygiene and the Bio-
    logical Action of Electromagnetic Fields of Superhigh Fre-
    quencies [in Russian], Meditsina.
Gordon, Z. V., Lobanova, E. A., and Tolgskaya, M. S., 1955, Gig.
    i San., 12:16.
Gorizontov, P. D., 1969, Abstracts of Proceedings of the 27th Ses-
    sion of the General Assembly of the Academy of Medical
    Sciences of the USSR on the Problem of "Current Endocri-
    nology and Hormone Biochemistry" [in Russian], Moscow.
Gorodetskaya, S. F., 1962, Fiziol. Zh. (Ukr.), 8(3):390.
Gorodetskaya, S. F., 1963, Fiziol. Zh. (Ukr.), 9:394.
Gorodetskaya, S. F., 1964, in: The Biological Action of Ultra-
    sound and Superhigh-Frequency Electromagnetic Waves
    [in Russian], Kiev, Naukova Dumka, p. 80.
Grashchenkov, N. I. (Editor), 1963, The Physiology and Pathology
    of the Diencephalic Region of the Brain [in Russian], Moscow,
    p. 5.
Grashchenkov, N. I., 1964, in: The Hypothalamus, Its Role in
    Physiology and Pathology [in Russian], Moscow.
Guillemin, R., 1961, Acta Neurovegetativa (Vienna), 23.
Guillemin, R., and Rosenberg, B., 1955, Endocrinology, Vol. 57.
Gunn, S., Gould, T., and Anderson, W., 1961, in: Biological Effects
    of Microwave Radiation, Plenum Press, New York, p. 99.
Gunn, S., et al., 1961, Lab. Invest., 10:301.
Guseinov, D. Yu., 1963, Arkh. Pat., No. 2, 45.
Howland, I., et al., 1961, in: Biological Effects of Microwave
    Radiation, Plenum Press, New York, p. 261.

Imig, C. L., Thomson, J. D., and Hines, H. M., 1948, Proc. Soc. Exp. Biol. (New York), 69(2):382.

Kitsovskaya, I. A., 1960, The Biological Effects of Superhigh Frequencies. Transactions of the Institute of Work Hygiene and Occupational Diseases, Academy of Medical Sciences of the USSR, No. 1, Moscow, p. 75.

Kitsovskaya, I. A., 1968a, in: Work Hygiene and the Biological Action of Radio Waves. Proceedings of the 3rd All-Union Symposium on June 24–28, Moscow, p. 71.

Kitsovskaya, I. A., 1968b, in: The Biological Action of Radio Waves. Transactions of the Institute of Work Hygiene and Occupational Diseases, Academy of Medical Sciences of the USSR [in Russian], No. 3, Moscow, p. 81.

Kulakova, V. V., 1968, in: The Biological Action of Radio Waves. Transactions of the Institute of Work Hygiene and Occupational Diseases, Academy of Medical Sciences of the USSR [in Russian], No. 3, Moscow, p. 112.

Kupriyanov, V. V., 1955, Material on the Experimental Morphology of Vascular Receptors [in Russian], Leningrad.

Kurlyandskii, B. A., 1966, Abstracts of Papers Read at a Toxicological Laboratory [in Russian].

Kurtsin, I. R. 1963, in: Cortico-Visceral Relationships and Hormonal Regulation [in Russian], Khar'kov.

Kutting, H., 1955, Med. Klin., 30:1262.

Lavrent'ev, B. I., 1934, Proceedings of the 1st Histological Conference [in Russian], Moscow.

Lavrent'ev, B. I. 1936, Fiziol. Zh. SSSR, 21(5–6):858.

Lavrent'ev, B. I., 1948, in: Morphology of the Sensory Innervation of the Internal Organs [in Russian], Izd. Akad. Med. Nauk SSSR.

Lazarev, N. V., 1963, Harmful Substances in Industry, Chapters I, II.

Levinson, A. B., 1952, Dokl. Akad. Nauk SSSR, 83(5):745.

Liebesny, P., 1936, Short and Ultrashort Waves. Biological Action [Russian translation], Moscow–Leningrad, p. 221.

Lobanova, E. A., 1960, in: The Biological Action of Radio Waves. Transactions of the Institute of Work Hygiene and Occupational Diseases, Academy of Medical Sciences of the USSR [in Russian], No. 1, Moscow, p. 61.

Lotis, V. M., 1936, Akush. i Gin., 10:1240.

Maiorova, V. F., 1962, Probl. Éndokrinol., Vol. 5.

Maiorova, V. F., and Tarakanov, E. I., 1964, Neurosecretory Elements and Their Role in the Organism [in Russian], Izd. AN SSSR.

Michaelson, S. M., et al., 1961a, Indust. Med. Surg., 30:298.

Michaelson, S. M., et al., 1961b, Digest Internat. Congr. Med. Electronics, 26:4.

Militsin, V. A., and Voznaya, A. I., 1937, Fizioterapiya, 2:33.

Milyutina, E. V., 1933, in: Data on the Biological Character of Ultrahigh-Frequency Radiation [in Russian], Gor'kii, p. 45.

Minecki, L., 1967, Promieniowanie Elektromagnetyczne wielkiey Czestotliwosci, Warsaw.

Minecki, L., and Bilski, P., 1961, Med. Pracy, 12(4):337.

Mosinger, M., 1950, Schweiz. Arch. Neurol. Psych., Vol. 65, Nos. 1/2.

Moskalenko, Yu. E., 1960, in: Electronics in Medicine [in Russian], Moscow—Leningrad, p. 207.

Mumford, W., 1961, Proc. IRE, 49:427.

Nikogosyan, S. V., 1964, in: The Biological Action of Radio Waves. Transactions of the Institute of Work Hygiene and Occupational Diseases, Academy of Medical Sciences of the USSR [in Russian], No. 2, Moscow, p. 43.

Nikonova, K. V., 1964, in: Biological Action of Radio Waves. Transactions of the Institute of Work Hygiene and Occupational Diseases, Academy of Medical Sciences of the USSR [in Russian], No. 2, Moscow, pp. 49 and 61.

Obrosov, A. N., and Yasnogorodskii, V. G., 1961, Abstracts of Proceedings of the 4th International Congress of Radioelectronics in Medicine, New York, p. 155.

Oettinger, 1931, Strahlentherapie, 41:251.

Orlova, A. A., 1960, in: Biological Action of Superhigh-Frequency Radiation. Transactions of the Institute of Work Hygiene and Occupational Diseases, Academy of Medical Sciences of the USSR [in Russian], No. 1, Moscow, p. 36.

Osipov, Yu. A., 1953, Sov. Zdravookhr., 2:44.

Parin, V. V., and Davydov, I. Ya., 1940, in: Problems in Physiotherapy and Balneology [in Russian], Sverdlovsk, p. 178.

Pervushin, V. Yu., 1957, Byull. Éksperim. Biol. i Med., No. 6, p. 87.

Pervushin, V. Yu., and Triumfov, A. V., 1957, in: The Biological Action of the Superhigh-Frequency Electromagnetic Field [in Russian], Leningrad, p. 141.

Pitenin, I. V., 1962, in: Problems in the Biological Action of a
    Superhigh-Frequency Electromagnetic Field [in Russian],
    Leningrad, p. 36.
Plechkova, E. K., 1948, in: The Morphology of the Sensory In-
    nervation of the Internal Organs [in Russian], Izd. Akad. Med.
    Nauk SSSR, pp. 163-179.
Polenov, A. L., 1964, Neurosecretory Elements and Their Role in
    the Organism [in Russian], Izd. AN SSSR.
Polyakov, G. I., 1955, Arkh. Anat. Gistol. i Émbriol., 32:2.
Polyakov, G. I., 1956, Zh. Vyssh. Nervn. Deyat., 6:3.
Porter, R. W., 1953, Am. J. Physiol., Vol. 172.
Porter, R. W., 1956, Endocrinology, Vol. 58.
Povzhitkov,V. A., et al., 1961, Byull. Éksperim. Biol. i Med., 51(5):103.
Presman, A. S., 1968, Electromagnetic Fields and Living Nature
    [in Russian], Nauka, Moscow.
Rakhmanov, A. V., 1940, Problems in the Use of Short and Ultra-
    short Waves in Medicine [in Russian], Moscow, p. 131.
Romasenko, V. A., 1967, Hypertoxic Schizophrenia [in Russian].
Sadchikova, M. N., and Orlova, A. A., 1958, Gig. Truda i Prof.
    Zabol., 1:16.
Sarkisov, S. A., 1948, Some Distinctive Structural Features of
    Interneuronal Connections in the Cerebral Cortex [in Russian],
    Moscow, Izd. Akad. Med. Nauk SSSR.
Scharrer, B., and Scharrer, E., 1954a, in: Handbuch der mikrosko-
    pischen Anatomie des Menschens, p. 13.
Scharrer, E., and Scharrer, B., 1954b, Recent Prog. Hormon. Res.,
    Vol. 10.
Schliephake, E., 1932, Kurzwellentherapie, Jena.
Selye, H., 1960, Essays on the Adaptation Syndrome [Russian trans-
    lation], Moscow.
Sequin, L., and Castelain, G., 1947, C. R. Acad. Sci., 224:1662 and
    1850.
Shibkova, S. A., 1937, Arkh. Anat. Gistol. i Émbriol., 17(1):72.
Skipin, G. V., and Baranov, N. P., 1934, Bulletin of the All-Union
    Institute of Experimental Medicine [in Russian], Leningrad,
    Vol. 3-4, p. 12.
Slavskii, G. M., and Burnaz, L. S., 1933, Transactions of the
    Sechenov Central Research Institute of Physiology [in Rus-
    sian], Sevastopol', Vol. 6-7, p. 294.
Smurova, E. I., 1962, Gig. Truda i Prof. Zabol., 5:22.

Spynu, E. I., 1959, Gig. i San., 11:26.

Syngaevskaya, V. A., Ignat'eva, O. S., Pliskina, T. P., and Sinenko, G. F., 1962, Abstracts of Proceedings of a Conference on the Biological Action of Superhigh-Frequency Radiation [in Russian], Leningrad, p. 52.

Tarakanov, E. I., Maiorova, V. F., et al., 1960, Probl. Éndokrinol. i Gormonoter., 6:3.

Tikhonova, M. A., 1948, in: Problems in Experimental Physiotherapy. Transactions of the N. A. Semashko Uzbek Research Institute of Physiotherapy and Balneology [in Russian], Tashkent, No. 10, p. 113.

Tolgskaya, M. S., and Gordon, Z. V., 1960, Biological Action of Superhigh Frequencies. Transactions of the Institute of Work Hygiene and Occupational Diseases, Academy of Medical Sciences of the USSR [in Russian], Leningrad, No. 1, p. 99.

Tolgskaya, M. S., and Gordon, Z. V., 1964, Biological Action of Radio Waves. Transactions of the Institute of Work Hygiene and Occupational Diseases, Academy of Medical Sciences of the USSR [in Russian], Moscow, No. 2, p. 80.

Tolgskaya, M. S., and Gordon, Z. V., 1968, Biological Action of Radio Waves. Transactions of the Institute of Work Hygiene and Occupational Diseases, Academy of Medical Sciences of the USSR [in Russian], Moscow, No. 3, p. 87.

Tolgskaya, M. S., Gordon, Z. V., and Lobanova, E. A., 1960a, in: Physical Factors of the External Environment [in Russian], Moscow, p. 183.

Tolgskaya, M. S., Gordon, Z. V., and Lobanova, E. A., 1960b, in: Biological Action of Superhigh Frequencies. Transactions of the Institute of Work Hygiene and Occupational Diseases, Academy of Medical Sciences of the USSR [in Russian], Moscow, No. 1, p. 90.

Tolgskaya, M. S., and Nikonova, K. V., 1964, in: The Biological Action of Radio Waves. Transactions of the Institute of Work Hygiene and Occupational Diseases, Academy of Medical Sciences of the USSR [in Russian], Moscow, No. 2, p. 89.

Ummersen, C., 1961, Proceedings of the 4th Annual Tri-Service Conference on the Biological Effects of Microwave Radiation, pp. 201-204.

Vladimirov, S. V., 1964, Neurosecretory Elements and Their Role in the Organism [in Russian], Izd. AN SSSR.

Voitkevich, A. A., 1964, Neurosecretory Elements and Their Role
    in the Organism [in Russian], Izd. AN SSSR.
Voitkevich, A. A., 1969, Abstracts of Proceedings of the 27th Ses-
    sion of the General Assembly of the Academy of Medical
    Sciences of the USSR on Problems in Modern Endocrinology
    and Hormone Biochemistry [in Russian], Moscow.
Vorotilkin, A. I., 1940, Problems in Physiotherapy and Balneology
    [in Russian], Sverdlovsk, p. 217.
Voznaya, A., and Sherdin, I., 1937, Transactions of the Institute
    of Physiotherapy and Physical Culture [in Russian],
    Moscow, No. 1, p. 48.
Zhdanov, D. A., Akmaev, I. G., and Sanin, M. R., 1964, Arkh. Anat.,
    No. 4.
Zhukhin, V. A., 1937, Transactions of the Turkmenian Research
    Institute of Neurology and Physiotherapy [in Russian], Ash-
    khabad, Vol. 2, p. 159.
Zhukova, S. V., 1964, Neurosecretory Elements and Their Role in
    the Organism [in Russian], Izd. AN SSSR.
Zubkova-Mikhailova, E. I., 1964, Neurosecretory Elements and
    Their Role in the Organism [in Russian], Izd. AN SSSR.